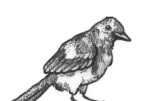

SONGS OF
FRIENDSHIP

**A
STORYTELLING
CYCLE**

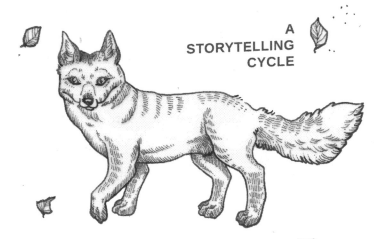

James Rowland

SONGS OF FRIENDSHIP

Team Viking

A Hundred Different Words for Love

Revelations

OBERON BOOKS
LONDON

WWW.OBERONBOOKS.COM

First published in 2018 by Oberon Books Ltd
521 Caledonian Road, London N7 9RH
Tel: +44 (0) 20 7607 3637 / Fax: +44 (0) 20 7607 3629
e-mail: info@oberonbooks.com
www.oberonbooks.com

A catalogue record for this book is available from the British Library.

PB ISBN: 9781786825339
E ISBN: 9781786825346

Cover illustrations by Wiggy Cheung

Printed and bound by 4EDGE Limited, Hockley, Essex, UK.
eBook conversion by Lapiz Digital Services, India.

Contents

Introduction

Two and a half years ago, an extremely hairy actor called James Rowland did what many performers have done before him: he asked everyone he knew to come and see a one-man show he had written and was starring in.

There was – possibly – probably – definitely – a collective sigh of premature resignation from those invited. Because there's supporting someone, and then there's indulging their enormous and fragile ego by sitting through an hour of them rambling on about shit in a damp room underground when you could be doing something nice and productive like sitting in a pub with natural light.

Just because you *can* ask lots of people in your life to volunteer as a literal captive audience to indulge your oral narrative whimsy doesn't mean you *should.*

But James knows many decent, kind, well-mannered souls all bound together by a fundamental inability to say 'no', and so he did.

However...

It was completely and utterly wonderful.

I have known James for nearly ten years.* As natural show-offs and would-be writer/performers, he and I bonded when we met on The Company Project in 2009. I liked his cherubic smile and penchant for cured meats; he liked my incredible body and shapely ankles.

What has followed since then has been a decade of loud (him), tender (me), loving and joyful friendship. We have helped each other through the full gamut of the human

---

* And I have enjoyed over 40% of our time together.

experience: falling in love, break-ups,* health scares, work triumphs, work disasters, burglaries, tax returns, and *Game of Thrones.*

I don't think I've ever felt prouder of the man, or more full of love for him, than when I watched him perform *Team Viking* for the first time at the Vaults Festival in 2016.† It (and he) genuinely took my breath away. Same again last year with *100 Different Words for Love*,‡ and then again a few months ago with *Revelations.*§ He possesses an uncanny ability to convey the warmth, humour and soaring joy that go hand-in-hand with the darkest, bleakest moments in all our lives: I have no doubt these plays will make make your heart sing, your eyes damp, and your bladder weak.

James is one of the kindest, funniest, cleverest, most generous people I have ever had the privilege to meet. I know we'll be friends until one of us dies.¶

This being true, I think we can safely assume *Songs Of Friendship* is about me.

I dedicate it to myself.

Charlie Covell, 2018

---

* When I was heartbroken, James gave me the unabridged *His Dark Materials* read by the actual Philip Pullman and a full cast. When he was heartbroken, I bought him a Groupon massage which he has only recently admitted was one of the more profoundly disappointing experiences of his life.

† He won the Origins Award for new writing for it.

‡ He won Show of The Year that time.

§ He didn't win anything this year.

¶ I gave up smoking before him.

To Lizzy Attwood, my mum.
Without whom, in every sense, I wouldn't be here.

TEAM VIKING

*

---

*   Hello. I'm being dreadfully transgressive right from the beginning by footnoting a blank page… Tread carefully as I am about to upturn every preconception you have ever had (unless you have one about my being amused by displays of faux-grandiosity.)

I'm doing footnotes because I personally don't love reading stuff that has been written to be performed. Also I've seen it work really well in Stewart Lee's *How I Escaped My Certain Fate* and the play texts for *Every Brilliant Thing* by Duncan Macmillan and Jonny Donahoe and *How To Win Against History* by Seiriol Davies.

Most importantly though, I was ill as a teenager so didn't get out much and Terry Pratchett's books stopped me from being totally miserable and that guy really knew how to use a footnote.

So I'm honouring all of them by bastardising their form.

You're welcome.

You don't have to read them if you don't want to.

Set: Stage right a microphone, loop pedal and Casio keyboard.

Upstage centre an old amp with a plastic Viking helmet and can of Lynx Africa sitting on it. *

A pre-amble, talking about the venue/weather/my health/the attractiveness of the audience (always positive regardless of my feelings). After clearance from front of house I ask if anyone has serious respiratory issues. †

I'm sure that you know that we perfume the bodies of the dead, Vikings did as well. Smell is also apparently the most potent of the senses when it comes to remembering.

> *I lightly spritz the audience with Lynx Africa unless someone has declared their asthma in which case I explain what would be otherwise happening.*

Now I'm going to go and do the lights and when I come back I will be a performer and all the rest of this will be artifice.‡

> *I go and dim the house lights.*§

---

*   The shows are just me with no stage manager or tech. This was initially for the very simple reason that I had no money to pay anyone but I think it became instantly useful in shaping the shows. Form bringing freedom; when you know what you can't do it prevents being paralysed by choice. I also get properly fucked off when I watch theatre where the bells and whistles are there for no real reason.

†   Bimbling around while the audience arrive seems to be integral to the shows. I guess it's relaxing. Also Dan likes it.

‡   All of the rest of these will be artifice as well. I know you're gonna read them, so how could they be anything but? It's all performance.

§   Depending on venue this can be rather different. *Team Viking* toured to theatres but also did a fair amount of rural touring which is generally small village halls without elaborate lighting rigs. There are rural touring networks all over the country, supported by the Arts Council and

Hello my name is James, I'm gonna tell you a story and all of it is true.*

I call upon Odin, King of the Gods and father of stories to aid me in this account.†

Music. ‡

---

donations. They are just wonderful, it's been a real pleasure and privilege to do this shows in communities. Whenever I do the show rurally I do a little speech before I crack on with the show taking about how regardless of political persuasion we can all agree that we are incredibly lucky to live somewhere where that sort of thing exists because art should be everywhere because it is for everyone.

I then moonwalk out of the building while the audience, bowled over by my wisdom and humility throw tributes at my glorious body.

* More on this later. Perhaps don't read the footnotes if you don't want this statement challenged.

† I can't remember where the invocation came from but it is a vital part of the shows. I'm such a furry, relaxed, amenable-looking person that adding an element of the epic at the start of the show stops people from forgetting that it is a show and we're not just chatting. Deliberately dissonant with the atmosphere created already.

‡ Throughout the show I make a song. Each musical break is one layer on the loop pedal. This first one is some simple chords on the Casio SA-46 on its 'brass' setting (number 47). I play it kneeling on the floor. This second odd thing following on from the relaxed opening tends to get a chuckle if the audience want to feel in control of the situation.

So.[*]

The sun was shining down; warm, not too hot, still and bright, *really bright;* like God had turned the contrast up on the world. Seeing the sharp, sharp edges of yourself and everything else. It wasn't just the light, I also had that cotton wool feeling, y'know, thick wads of cotton wool insulating you and at the same time you're observing things more than usual because of the awareness of separation between yourself and the outside world and...

People were milling about, lots of people, so many people, I think there were eight hundred or something; more people than I could be friends with or know, and I was grief-handing which is like glad handing but at a sad time, 'Hi nice to –' 'University, I see –' 'Yeah, yeah, yeah,' 'Thank you my speech was very good' (I didn't say that obviously), but people were being, Dad's old friends they were being very kind, they said that what I said was good, I think one of them described it as profoundly moving, which I found profoundly gratifying.

It was lovely, I s'pose. In fact there were so many people there that all of Dad's old students had to go in the church hall, the overflow, they'd set up some sort of audio relay so they could hear the whole ceremony, my speech.[†]

---

[*] The word 'so' seems to be very useful to solo storytelling. George Perrin pointed this out to me when we rehearsed *Every Brilliant Thing.* I hadn't noticed that I'd already used it loads in this and *A Hundred...* but I think it's because it works as active punctuation that keeps a story travelling.

[†] This whole scene is entirely based on the funeral of a teacher I had at Drama School. Mr Hall was a wonderful man, inspiring, gentle and kind. Capable of turning a boring day into a great one. I was incredibly lucky to become friends with him before he died. It felt right to make it my Dad's funeral to make the impact more immediate and active.

It's great at a funeral, if you can hold it together (obviously not emotionally, let that shit* out), but if you don't think you're a funny person and you want to do a joke and have people laugh, just save it for a funeral, or when someone's suffering from the profound effects of grief because it makes people really susceptible, you can do anything, knock-knock jokes, funny noises, even mime, people will love it. I'd done all three – yeah my speech was pretty weird. There I was in the aftermath, people milling around, lost in my own hazy daze.

Tom and Sarah approach, Tom a proud peacock.[†]

'Great speech mate –' (course he'd say that he helped me write it) '– shame about the delivery.'

'...'

Sarah: 'It was great, you did him proud.'

'I'm going over there now,' Tom, motioning to a group of my Dad's old students.

---

* You may notice that I am not shy of a swear. I think words are words and swear words are just another way of expressing ourselves. However, I also know that that is just my opinion so if I get the sense that the audience might be put off by f-ing and blinding[†] I cut all of the casual curses out and hold them back for the significant emotional moments.

† fucking and blinding[‡]

‡ I do not blind anyone[§]

§ footnotes to footnotes!

† This scene is the first bit of 'acting'. Tom always had a very clearly different physicality and voice from me. Sarah on the other hand is much more subtly different and as a result she seemed less real for a long time then one day it was just working despite no obvious change in the performance.

Sarah: 'He's pretending to be you to try and pull.'

Tom: 'They're really pretty Jim, besides, it's what your old man would have wanted.'*

Sarah, lighting a cigarette, 'Sure, but is it what they want?'

Tom, on his way, 'Absolutely.'

We laugh.

Sarah assesses my face.

'You okay Jim?'

'…'

and she gives me a hug, one of those glorious world-beating hugs where you realise what a weight you've been carrying because it's not there in that instant.

Tom and Sarah my best friends since…forever. We grew up together, the three of us, in a suburban, middle class, middle England – there was nothing middling about it though because it was fucking extraordinary. Of course now I've grown up, I've seen a lot more of the world and I understand that so much of it was this privileged idyll, surrounded by enough money for a lot of imagination, but you see, we were the last generation who played outside, and looking back on us now I understand why people really push the computers because if all the other kids are like we were. I'm very happy they're sat inside quietly glued to a screen because:

---

* Tom really did this at Mr Hall's funeral.

'Oh look there's a window, oh and here are some stones...
hey guys I've just thought of the best game!'* Yeah, we were
dangerous. We were so dangerous we got banned from
reading the Just William books because we did too many of
the things in them.† So watch out.

I met Tom first, when we were very young (we went to the same
crèche and stuff) his mum was on her own, so he used to come
over to our house when she went out on dates. Which was quite
a lot. A very organised lady in a pre-internet dating world.

We played Knights, we played Robin Hood but mostly and
most importantly we played Vikings. Inspired by the 1958
film with Kirk Douglas and Tony Curtis.‡ Has anyone seen
it? It's amazing isn't it? And it exploded like a glorious atom
bomb in our nascent consciousnesses.

The story of Vikings is this: you have Kirk Douglas, blond hair,
bum chin, he is Prince Einar, the anti-hero. His likes include:
quaffing, wenching and fighting. His dislikes: everything else.
Total Viking. Then there's Tony Curtis, honest faced, wearing
only a beard, a burning sense of justice and some historically

---

*   Genuinely played this game once when I was a kid. Got in so much trouble.

†   Also true.

‡   Never saw it until I made this show. Despite this being a true story I took
a lot of liberties with real events to make the story more dramatic and
also in some cases more real. It seemed totally unbelievable that any of
this would have happened without there being some big emotional tie
to Vikings. Dan introduced me to this movie when we were making the
show and it filled the gap perfectly. If we had actually been inspired by
childhood heroes it would have been Robin Hood's death we imitated.
I feel like firing an arrow out of a UCLH window and burying Tom
wherever that landed would have been even more bizarre than the events
in this story.

inaccurate very revealing leather hot pants, he is Erik, the illegitimate son of the English Queen and the Viking King, Erik the bastard, our hero. Then there's a princess that both of our boys are in love with, eye gouging hawks, flesh eating crabs, man eating wolves (nature is all very dangerous in Vikings) castles being scaled, evil Kings – it's got everything.

I would always be Einar because blond hair, bum chin before the beard and Tom: Erik the bastard cos No Dad...* and from the age of four or five you would find us conquering the castles of England in the drizzle of our back-gardens on a daily basis. It was great fun.†

Enter Sarah, from over the fence next door. Perfect, we needed a princess to ravish.

'Would you like to play with us?'

'That depends. What are you playing?'‡

'Vikings, have you seen it?'

'Don't think so.'

Fast forward two hours later –

'So that was pretty great.'

---

* The ellipses here represents the pause I have to leave here for an audience laugh that always happens (hubris) to welcome the first proper joke in the show. Everyone tends to relax after this, although maybe that's just me.
† I know that we rose tint the past but that's fine with me. My memories of playing in our little gardens are of pure happiness.
‡ I have absolutely no memory of what Sarah was like as a child but I like to imbue her with as much poise and sang-froid as possible here. Even more than my impression of her often poker faced adult self.

'Yep. So you can be the Princess –'

'I'm not going to be her. She's boring. I'll be Eric.'

Tom made it clear that that was not gonna happen, over his dead body.

'In that case, I'll be the other one, Einar.'

'But I'm Einar.'

'Probably not anymore,' was their consensus.

So from then on I would be the dangerous animals, or the castle, or the beautiful princess (I was a wonderful beautiful princess). Whatever was necessary to keep the narrative spinning because we just had to do the whole film over and over.

We could only do the final scene one time though (cos our special effects budget was quite small). We got my paddling pool filled up, Playmobile pirate ship, covered in twigs and set ablaze with my gerbil Ragnar on board. Best. Day. Ever.

It's important to point out that Ragnar was dead already, we weren't psychopaths.*

And that was the beginning of Tom, Sarah and me. We were Team Viking.

---

* This didn't happen. For a start, I didn't have a Playmobile pirate ship and if I had had one it would have been far too valuable a commodity to set fire to. I never cremated a gerbil. Did get my dog drunk on Baileys once though which I think is worse.

I had a drag of Sarah's cigarette, made more small talk with strangers, watched Tom get not one but two numbers and in his words a 'cheeky goodbye kiss' and whsssh, everyone vanished, I've never seen eight hundred people disappear so quickly, we went to the crematorium, weird sad music played something woefully inappropriate, the curtains closed. The curtains closed and that was that. We went for dinner (Pizza Express obviously) my family, Tom, Sarah, my girlfriend Esther, lest I forget, she'd been there, she'd been with my mum all day, she'd been great. The next day I had to come back to London – the pub had only given me a few days off. Sarah gave me a lift (I had a train ticket but she was coming back to continue her PhD at Imperial so she drove).

Mum kept the Ashes, I still don't know what she did with them – I should probably ask...

*Music.**

Back down in London, I just carried on in a sort of mechanical way. Funny thing about machines: they're not very good at relationships, but I had computed that Esther was sad, and I calculated that that was because I was sad, so I thought we'd do a lovely thing, try and press restart: go to Victoria Park, hire a rowing boat and go out on the lake. Romantic. Then the guy running the boats was a real prick for no reason,

---

* This is sung. A open Ah following the tune in the middle of my register... I'm becoming aware that describing music with words is frankly fucking terrible. Sorry. I'll put them up online at some point so you can listen to them.

it's not like his job's shit – so just be kind alright and if you can't be kind be nice. But no, he was an arse about me not having the right change, then when we did get a boat one of the oars was split – and he was just *so rude* it was a relief when Esther suggested we just sack the whole thing off and go back to her place.

So we went back to her house and she broke up with me.

Two days later, getting home from a day shift at the pub. Tom and Sarah sitting on my doorstep. Ooof, so fucking nice, oh yeah, apparently Esther had called Sarah and said, 'Just so you know, I've broken up with James, I don't think he's gonna be alright, so maybe you guys should…' Nice, right? But before you think that she's really cool and awesome for doing that, you should know that she broke up with me by metaphor. In her bedroom (that I helped decorate), surrounded by the innumerable throw pillows, she was like:

I would now approach the audience and quickly ask to borrow some bags and coats. I'd then target a man in the front row.

So you're me and I'm Esther.

I then pile the audience belongings on him one by one.

'You see James, a little bit of love is nice

but when there's too much love

and too many things

you just feel stifled.'

23

...I stayed like that for ages. About another forty minutes.*

Essentially she broke up with me with a GCSEs drama project. Anyway, that didn't matter because Tom and Sarah were down so we were going out.†

And it was one of the great nights. We went to the same places we always went, told the same stories, played the same games but you know that thing where it just clicks? We were golden, you couldn't touch us. Tom was in the middle of it all of course. Drunk as anything but right on it. If you didn't know Tom you might think he had a drink problem or a drugs problem, whatever, he had a fucking *solution*. The more he drank the more he radiated this anarchic joy, casting his spell on anyone who came close.

So. It gets to closing time at the King's Head in London: the city that always sleeps at midnight, but that wasn't gonna stop us, that wasn't stopping Tom, or Sarah, or James. No fuck that, we're going to the Dolphin in Hackney that never closes!‡ And we won't go by taxi, or by bus, no, we'll go by

---

* This really happened. Someone broke up with me exactly like this. I have changed their name to protect the very, very guilty BUT to be fair I'd definitely break up with me too.
  Jenny Chiodini. Her name is Jenny Chiodini. Hi Jenny.
† This bit ramps up the energy in the show. It's the first acceleration of intensity that very slowly crescendoes through the first third of the show, hopefully imperceptible to the audience. Like boiling a frog. Hot water everywhere.
‡ The Dolphin is so popular that just mentioning it gets a cheer with some audiences. I once poured two full candles over my naked chest while performing an interpretative dance version of *Born to Run* there. I mention it because there's a good chance that that was the best performance I will ever give and I want that recorded.

Camel Race (which is exactly like a piggy back race but just better because camels are better than pigs).* I had Sarah on my back, Tom some random medical student in a penguin onesie on his. We were followed by a badger carrying a zebra, a Dalmatian carrying a panda with a skunk (obviously on their own) bringing up the rear, a monochrome ark-load of future doctors with our Noah – Tom leading the way.

When suddenly he tripped. Hit the ground hard and was just staying down – she was fine, the penguin, just dusting herself off – but Tom had gone down hard and was just. Staying. Down... By the time we'd got to him though he was up, grinning, blood trickling from the new holes in his trousers and shouting 'Kiss chase!' through his grimace. So we had to get as far away as possible, fast.

Tom. One in a million.

Oh as a sidebar, just a quick piece of advice, if you have children, now or in the future, obviously you can't make them do anything, but do encourage them to grow up through childhood and adolescence in a mixed group of friends, girls and boys. It makes those teenage years so much easier. I mean, admittedly all our formative sexual experiences were with each other and looking back on that I would rather lose my eyes than ever do any of it again but I think it was healthy, for us at least, I think. We've grown up relatively happy and

---

* This as I'm sure you have noticed isn't particularly funny and doesn't make much sense. Instead of trying to fix that, at some point I decided that I like the fact that I'm having fun and no one else is, so much so that sometimes the audience get into it. Could have just said piggy backs.

25

well-adjusted together and now I fancy girls, Tom has sex with all the things (he's omnisexual) and Sarah is an engineer…

I mean you're right it was a more innocent time in those halcyon days, no high-speed internet back then, no no, we found our pornography in hedges, I mean we didn't know why the hedges were making it, we were just glad that somebody was and grateful for that education.*

Anyway, we got to the Dolphin, everyone had a ball and it got to the natural lull time, three/four in the morning, sitting outside smoking, the penguin Tom had been kissing waddled off home.

Sarah sitting between us. Tom grabbed me over the table. 'Look, I just wanted to say I'm really sorry about your dad's funeral.'

I was like 'What? You weren't a prick, you were fine.'

'I know that mate I'm a fucking legend, no what I'm saying is that is not what a funeral should be, all those people but no letting go, it was just funeral foreplay.'

'So what? A piss-up so everyone could cry together? Funerals cost a lot already.'

'I know mate, 3,600 pounds is the average and that doesn't include a headstone –'

'How'd you know that?'

---

* This feels like the sort of idea/joke that loads of people must have made before. I'm lucky to be friends exclusively with very clever, original comics who would never stoop to making such a basic, nostalgia-driven joke. So I can do it because I've never seen anyone else.

'Doesn't matter. No, what I'm saying is it should be about catharsis, sharing properly.'

'So what would you suggest?'

'Your dad was a fucking big guy –'

(He'd been a bit of a surrogate to Tom, a strong male presence that I don't think is necessary but in the 2.4 children world we grew up in, I think it was maybe useful to have someone filling that societal space for him. In some ways Tom was more like Dad than I was, larger than life.)

'– he should have been like Einar –'

That's a spoiler, because Kirk Douglas dies at the end of *Vikings*. You've had seventy years to watch it. He gets the full works though, longship covered in logs, drums beating it onto the open ocean as a flaming arrow follows it there. It's amazing.

'I mean why not? Your dad deserved that, why not?'

'Well, for a start, I think you're fundamentally misunderstanding what funer– '

(At that point my state of inebriation was such that there was no way I'd be able to pronounce the words fundamentally, misunderstanding, or indeed inebriation but that's the wonder of editorialising isn't it.)

'– funerals are about, they're for the people who are still there, not the people who have gone.'

'No listen Jimbo, it's like – look you know how we've agreed that when we get married we'll all be best men for each other –'

Sarah interjected at this point. '– best men of honour.'

'Exactly! Well this is even bigger, giving each other the send-off we deserve, I mean why not?'

'Well for a start I think you're conflating* two entirely different things, weddings and funerals.'

'No Jim you're not listening, it's like Tim and Tara's wedding – after they left what did we do?'

'We stayed and partied.'

'Exactly. The people who we were there for had gone but that didn't stop us celebrating them and when I go, I want you guys to do something huge, something memorable, something that people'll tell stories about.'

'Again I just don't think that's what funerals –'

'You know fuck you Jimbo, if you carry on like this, I'll drag you to the park and give you the funeral you deserve right now.'

(Which is apparently a shallow grave covered in dog poo.)†

Sarah laughed. 'He makes a solid point, Jim.'

So I agreed. We all agreed and that was that. The next day Tom went home. Sarah vanished back to the lab (or whatever it is that she does) and I slipped back into my routine. We were meant to see each other at Christmas because we always saw each other at Christmas but that year, with Dad gone,

---

* I usually literally wink at the audience here calling back to the bit about editorialising. What a cheeky chappy.
† The line was 'dog shit' until I did a show where I toned down the swearing and poo is definitely funnier than shit.

Mum had decided we'd go to her parents' down in Devon and Devon is a long way away from...anywhere.*

So that was that. A boring, normal, mundane family Christmas – except for one thing, and you're gonna hear it cos it was brilliant. Mum had done the whole Christmas dinner, everything, all the trimmings in her parents' house. Grandma had only done the Christmas pudding, that was her one contribution so there was going to be a ceremony attached to it.

Grandpa master of said ceremony.

He had everything he needed; a half bottle of brandy, a little cup to pour it into, a box of matches and Parkinson's.†

Thing about Parkinson's is it makes it very easy to light matches – but very, very, hard to keep them lit. He poured the brandy into the cup, sprinkled it on the pudding, then took a match...and lit...and out, and another lit and out, and lit and out... Grandma at his elbow whispering, 'For goodness sake John, get it lit.' Grandpa in his own little world having a lovely time, concentrating. Mum and I exchanging glances, 'Well we could obviously help but this is their thing, this is their thing,' and lit and out and lit and out... Until he finally got one touched to the pudding, by which time the brandy had

---

* I'm not sure why I decided to throw shade at Devon but it went down incredibly well in Dorset and no one else cares.

† First joke about a horrible disease in the show. I find it tough that, in making jokes that can in a small way alleviate the mind-shattering heartbreak of being alive, it's impossible not to upset some people. This is the only line I've had a complaint about and I think the complaint was fair. But so is the joke.

just soaked through so the whole thing had to be started again. Brandy into the cup, on the pudding, matches, and lit and out and lit and out and lit and out... 'John, if the neighbours hear about this they'll be laughing down their sleeves at us they really will!' And more matches and more brandy, Mum and me gripping hands under the table, white-knuckled, holding on, 'Don't laugh, don't laugh this is brilliant don't laugh.' Grandpa in the zone, making a little wood pile under the matchbox and more brandy, and more matches and more brandy. 'They will publish a report in the *Gazette*, we will be pariahs!' Mum and I in a silent Munchian scream of agonised joy. And more matches and more brandy and more matches and more brandy and more brandy until finally, he got one touched to the pudding in time and 'WUMPPHH' the thing fucking exploded and there was this biblical pillar of fire in the middle of the dining room table because it would not go out.

Grandma looking from the scorch mark on the ceiling to the smoke alarm and back again, mollified slightly when the smoke alarm went off, Mum completely helpless, I fell off my chair (which I thought was something that only happens in stories). Grandpa the only person with his shit together. Very slow shit though, as he took himself off to the kitchen, got a damp cloth, came back and laid it over the now entirely charcoaled Christmas pudding. More out of respect than anything else. 'Don't look at it. It's too sad.'*

---

* This is a crucial comic set piece and it was absolutely terrible for absolutely ages. I didn't really work out how to do it until halfway through Edinburgh and I think a fair amount of that was to do with confidence, the rest of it was pace and not using good words, I dunno. It's important because as Robbie Williams said, 'You've gotta get high before you taste the lows.'

You see? Worth it.

Anyway, that was the only remarkable thing that happened to me the entire winter.

So it's February and Sarah calls me* – she's been speaking to Grace, Tom's mum.

Tom is ill, he's really ill.

At first the doctors thought it was blood pressure, a heart murmur, a slowing down...enough to stop him doing all the things he did. Turns out though that Tom is one in more than a million, maybe one in more than a hundred million aged twenty-five because Tom is going to die of a primary cardiac angiosarcoma.

Cancer of the heart.

It is so rare it's very hard to pick up on, and it's a death sentence. Instances of survival do not exist.

You don't get any time, three-six months, bish, bash, bosh.

Music.†

Cardiac angiosarcoma. That's what he had. I thought back to the night at the Dolphin and wondered if... No way of knowing though.

---

*   This was a very bad phone call.

†   This music is very low 'ooh-ing' then at the end a low 'let's die idiots together'.

So as the big mamma bear of the NHS lumbered into life to try and do the impossible, Tom's befuddled pigeons flocked to ease the inevitable. There is a specialist at UCLH who's as good as it gets with rare cancers, so Tom crashed at my place until a bed became free. His mum Grace (I should say by the way – forget nominative determinism, whatever you think when you hear the word Grace she is the opposite, there is nothing graceful about her at all*) had friends that only lived a few streets away from the hospital and she could stay with them so that was fine. Sarah took a sabbatical and we braced ourselves, all four of us in it together. We were going to be there, and we were going to watch Tom go.

On the first day of this chemo we were all ready, together, waiting, it felt weird though – small room, cramped, too many of us, so Sarah and I left them to it. Went to a pub over the road, sat, nursing a pint between us and making up cancer jokes. Tumor humour. It grows on you. Cut it out? I can't, it's inoperable and I'm malignant...†

I got a call, must be Grace because it was Tom's number that came up but it was *Tom* on the phone.

'Mate, I am outside, can you come round the corner coz I'm trying to stay out of sight of the hospital.'

He was there: hiding behind the pub blackboard, dressing-gowned, still plugged in, holding his drip bag on his shoulder,

---

* It is a testament to what a wonderful woman she is that after watching the show, Grace was not upset that I had painted her to be a nightmare for comic effect and the narrative of the story.

† These *incredible* puns get a very mixed response.

woozy as hell and intent on having a drink with us like a *nightmare made flesh*. So I panicked, I'm a human. Sarah thought it would be interesting to see if he got served. WHICH HE DID?!* He could only have a little bit of his pint[†] though because he was really on edge, and so we helped him up back to his hospital room. Where Grace was incandescent and made the lives of one or two nurses a living hell for a while. Tricky, but I was relieved she wasn't pointed in my direction.

Obviously Tom was being a completely reckless idiot but there is a salient point there if you look for it. Which is hospitals don't get to do what they want with you, they get to do what you want with you...obviously they know better about all of the health implications and stuff, they've got Google, but you're not discharged from hospital, you discharge yourself. They don't own you, unless you're sectioned for your own safety or the safety of those around you, in which case there'll be some paperwork that you'll probably notice.[‡]

Of course they are doing what they're doing for our good and it's one of the most glorious gifts that anyone gives to anyone in this difficult world: the gift of *health*. But I think it's so important to remember at those times, the hard times,

---

* The Northumberland Arms by Warren Street Station is not unused to selling alcohol to patients from UCLH. I became friends with one of Tom's nurses and we went for a drink there but had to leave as four of her patients had escaped and she didn't want to deal with them.

† It turns out that some types of chemotherapy are actually fine with alcohol... Not the stuff Tom was on though. Oh well, you live and learn. Or not.

‡ Depending on how the show is going here I add a bit along the lines of: 'Unless you're my Uncle Tim, who was too far gone.'

the worst times, that you always have control over what care to accept, you always have control over your*self.* *

All through that time Tom really enjoyed pretending that he had caught cancer from my dad, cue a lot of exasperated medical professionals[†] trying pointlessly and for ages to explain that 'that's not how it works'. He was delighted after several weeks' concerted lobbying to be allowed to try his first ever Brompton Cocktail (an archaic mix of cocaine and morphine, and I'm sure delicious in any circumstance that you're not allowed to have it.[‡]) Like I say though, it worked fast,[§] cardiac angiosarcomas are quick. He deteriorated rapidly and we were there taking shifts. Which was amazing of the nurses because obviously visiting hours wouldn't have allowed it, but they understood, so either Grace or Sarah or me[¶] would stay over.

Because it was getting to that point, and I'm sure that some of you will know what I mean. There's a point of no return with cancer, a point where the pain and the drugs are too much

---

* This whole thought is entirely indebted to Terry Pratchett's Richard Dimbleby Lecture (available on YouTube) on assisted dying.

† We experimented with 'Junior Doctors' here which weirdly got a bigger laugh. This could also be a perfect instance of Dan suggesting a better line than I had come up with and me being stubborn and self-defeating and saying no for no particular reason.

‡ While on some incredibly strong doses of opiates, Tom was not given the medical equivalent of a speedball. He did ask for it though. I suppose I'm indulging him in some fun after the fact.

§ Sometimes when I'm a bit loose here the audience laugh because they think I'm still talking about semi-recreational drug use.

¶ This deliberate grammatical mistake is a plant for later. I'm clever. Sooooo clever. I'm so clever I quite often forget to say it wrong which takes a fair amount of weight away from the pay-off.

for the sufferer to stay themselves, and you know that's the beginning of the end... Just before that though, a few days maybe...there's a funny thing that people seem to know, the mind being aware of the body or some sort of force of will keeping the sufferer going. So, so many people die having had some sort of closure or catharsis for their life. It might be something flippant but it is important, I want to be clear, I'm not saying that a positive mental attitude will stop a body dissolving – death and taxes right?* But so many people hold on for some sort of finale, whether it's something in the ether or a subconscious eye for detail that belies our day to day sensitivity.

With Tom it was very simple, he would not stop going on about the Dolphin agreement.

'You promised.'

Sarah was having none of it.

'Tom, it's not gonna be about you anymore. Of course it's about you now but when we get there it's got to be about Grace, about what she wants and she needs.'

'Oh come on. Jim, surely you understand?'

'Sorry mate, I agree with Sarah, your mum is going through enough without all of us losing our minds on top of everything else.'

---

* 'And I'm pretty sure that these days you can just not pay your taxes,' is an optional joke here. This whole bit is very sad because it is directly asking people to think about anyone they have lost to cancer. Sometimes the relief is welcome, other times it feels important to keep it still.

'It's not about her, not about her at all, it's about us, it's about what we promised, together, as friends.'

'It's not though is it mate, because if it was about that you wouldn't be talking to us, you know we'll do anything for you, you know we will. It's about your mum. If you thought it could really happen you'd be talking to her.'

'Fuck you Jim, you're only saying that because you're afraid, you're a fucking coward, you don't care enough.'

'No, mate, actually, and that's really unfair. This is just so silly... Because we know it never even happened like that anyway. It's just like the horns on Viking helmets – they never had horns on their helmets.* It's just another thing made up by movies and by storytellers, made up by people who thought that it sounded good.'†

'Yeah, well it wasn't made up when we were kids was it Jim. We knew it was real.'

That's the thing about stories – they can be better than real life.

I'm sure you know Odin's messengers are the ravens, so I can only imagine that he had arranged for a paint job because

---

* Vikings didn't have horned helmets. Probably. Someone told me that they found one recently but I can't remember who told me and I don't know who the 'they' who are supposed to have found it are. So. Vikings didn't have horns on their helmets. The myth began with the Romantics doing what they did best and romanticising stuff. Ah, horns. Romantic.

† The publicity for the show all read: 'A while ago my best friend Tom died of heart cancer. His last wish was for a Viking burial. So I gave him one.' But the show never explicitly states that that is what is at stake. Is it being unspoken a fun game? Is it wilful obtuseness? I mean it's both but I also think it keeps people interested.

all through that time I kept on seeing solitary magpies watching me.*

One for sorrow.

One for sorrow.

One for sorrow.

Music.†

One morning at the hospital. Grace had gone back to her friends', she'd stayed over. Me and Sarah were both there (Sarah and I were also both there depending on what sort of an idiot you are‡) and Tom asked to be sat up with the magic elevator bed:§

---

* This began as homage to my favourite joke of all time. Tom Bell's 'magpies' joke. I decided the best way to honour it was to use the same structural materials but make it really miserable. Tom Bell rarely performs stand-up anymore as a result of doing telly and film 'acting'. Which is a shame.

† This is the one where I do the lyrics:
This probably isn't a good idea
We're all idiots for being here
But the world makes little sense at all
Why try and change the weather
So let's sing on through all the shit
And let's die idiots together

‡ Is it a joke? Is it a dig at people who think that the sanctity of the rules of grammar are more important than fresh and vivid use of whatever symbols or sounds we have to express the knotted wonder behind our eyes? It's trying to be both.

§ At some point on the tour I realised this was a great opportunity for a physical joke. Tom slowly being sat up with a 'vvvvvvvvmm' noise, being about to speak then 'vvvvvmm' back down, over and over. It's fun to try

37

'I just want to speak to you both separately, I need to talk to you both individually.'

Bit odd. Ever the gentleman I let Sarah go first (because I needed a wee), did what I had to do, waited in the hallway, watched the clock ticking over, listened to the receptionists chatting away, looked out of the window – way, way down in the car park there was some horrible accident on the corner people running around –

Sarah came out. She was not good; eyes leaking, and she just looked at me with this pity, clearly so sorry, I mean I don't know why but why look at me like that, obviously it made me really keen to get on in there, really looking forward to what he had to say.

So I went in. Sat down. Looked at the shadow of my friend and waited for him to start.

'Y'see Jim, I had a thought about things, which is: I've never been one for FOMO, I've always danced away from it, made where I am the place people have fear of missing out for, but this is it, this is what it feels like, I am going to miss out on a shit-ton of things now.'

Pretty on the nose. What else is even the most flippant bit of Fear Of Missing Out other than our awareness that our lives are short and we could maybe be enjoying ourselves better somewhere else. Having a better time with this fraction of our fractional lives.* YOLO. (That means you only live once – I can never tell.)

---

and string it out as long as possible. The more ill Tom is and the more difficult he finds it to start speaking the funnier audiences seem to find it.

* I realised that if I do it slowly this is a great opportunity to be present in

'So that's the joke bit... Oh Jim, I just, I know that you've told me, I know you're not gonna give – do what I want you to – and maybe with your dad it was the right thing, a compromise that left no one unhappy...but I need you to do this for me – whether you can square it away with Mum or whether you can find some other way around it, cos. The fact is James. I fucking love you.'

'Oh mate I love you too –'

'No, no, that's not what I'm saying. I'm saying I'm in love with you, you dick... I have been in love with you I think since I've been able to feel that way.

I just think that if you could just do this, just do...some big romantic gesture – maybe that could make up for some of the years – all this time... Sarah just promised she'd help.'

What could I say to that?

I couldn't say yes. I said yes.

I mean, I had no intention of doing anything of the sort because when he's dead he's dead.* But what could I say?

Having got what he wanted he went on:

---

the room inviting the audience to run free and go and make the most of life. To kiss and hold those close to them. No one has ever done so which I assume to mean that every audience so far either have perfect lives or are cowards. I'm sure at some point someone will take the chance to just get away from me and I'll have to try to sell it as the beginning of a revolution to a jaded audience who have seen through my bullshit.

* I often don't say the second 'he's dead' and just imply it with a pause. Is this footnote even worth writing? Are any of them? Please don't tell me, I'm having fun.

'I'm aware that this might put up some sort of a barrier between us for the rest of this but I need you to know Jim I'm not in any shape to have sex with you at the moment, and if I was to have sex I'd probably do it with Paula (one of the nurses). Again. Because she was really gentle and knew what to do with me last time."*

I went out. A long, wordless hug with Sarah. Then at arm's length, red-eyed, she smiled painful:

'Well at least it can't get any fucking worse.'

I left, stumbled out of the hospital. Floating in my own bleary bubble. I got on the tube, trembling, full of a blur of emotion. Unaware of everyone else. Confused, no, not confused, I dunno. I mean, what the f– how can you? I dunno. I didn't know. It was a lot, it was too much. Oh. Dizzy with the fucking pointlessness. It just felt so wrong. I mean how dare he, how dare he put that on me, actually. How could he feel that, how could his feelings be so different? I was sitting on the end of a row, which is not the right thing to do on the tube, and an old lady got on but I didn't notice, I was too busy wrapped up in my solipsistic grief celebrity to care about anyone else but she must have got on, she must have got on because she fell over my legs on her way to an empty seat so there was I just the worst person in the entire world – WE NEVER HAD ANY SECRETS.

Sorry. That was a lot. I'm still angry…because we never had any secrets, the three of us. We never – it was too much.

---

* Tom really said this when he was days away from dying. I'm pretty sure he was joking. Pretty sure.

Too much.

Just this one thing, opening the floodgates, and there I was:
drowning in the enormity of everything.

Music. [*]

I got a phone call from Sarah when I got back home.[†] She
sounded totally hysterical.[‡]

'What's up mate?'

'Oh James, it's awful. It's so awful. I know I'm laughing but
it's terrible, you're not going to believe it, it's funny, it's so
terrible it's funny.'

'Just tell me what's happening?'

'Okay, but first you have to promise not to hate me because
I am going to laugh but it is terrible.'

'What's going on?'

'Grace got run over by an ambulance.'

---

[*] I make the decision to go to the mic but can't sing so instead beat out a
drum rhythm on the microphone. And cut out the song on 'let's die –'

[†] The rest of this story is entirely fictitious, action-wise. I felt almost all of
the feelings though.

[‡] Using the word hysterical to describe the emotional state of a woman is
dangerous. My friend Lizzy says: 'The problem with the word hysterical
is that it is used whenever women show emotion and is intrinsically
feminine.' That is the word I've said every time I've done the show though
which is why it's printed. I'm a work in progress.

Yeah, when she left us, the thing I'd seen out of the window. The accident on the corner of the car park. She'd left, she hadn't slept, she was exhausted, she didn't look, she didn't look and it hit her and she was gone and she was dead. Just bounced her head off the curb and died before it had reversed back to her...

I mean you'd think it'd be the ideal way to get hit wouldn't you? I mean if you're going to get hit by a vehicle what sort would you like it to be? And how close would you like to be to a hospital, still in the car park or further? But ambulances are heavy and it doesn't matter how close you are to a hospital when your brain isn't inside your head anymore and it's just smeared on the pavement.*

---

* SO. Grace is very much alive and well and living in the West Country but I killed her (in the story, this isn't an elaborate confession). When she came to see the show she was a little annoyed at being killed off. I explained as best I could.

The process of making the shows involves making lots of decisions in the moment. When I did the first improv of this for Dan after months of thought, research and vacillation, I set up the story as if Grace was an obstacle to fulfilling Tom's wishes because there has to be conflict. I got about halfway through and realised as I was talking that there was no satisfying way of quickly wrapping that up. This is a story about a tragic young death seen through the lens of friendship rather than family. So I just said out of nowhere, 'Then Grace died,' and continued to talk while Daniel laughed for ages. It's so shocking that it seems true and I don't think audiences would buy the rest of the show in the same way without it. What possible reason would I have for making up something so horrible after all? Taking the path of a compulsive liar: tell such big, pointless lies that it seems stupid to disbelieve them.

Subsequently it was very hard to unlock the comedy in it again until Charlie suggested that Sarah should find it funny. It's easier for the audience to laugh at the horror of it if it's not me suggesting it's amusing.

So Grace was dead, and the question was: how do we tell Tom? Do we what? Do we hmmm.

Let's workshop that:

'Mate, how you feeling – don't answer that. Right. I've got some good news and some bad news.'

…

'The good news? You're not going to die before your mum.'

No, thankfully a scene to be theorised by science fiction writers, because after our chat that morning… Well, that's when he went off a cliff – that's when he passed the point of no return. His life was over and his death had begun.

So he couldn't be at his mum's funeral (a crematorium in Wood Green), but that was okay because no one else could either. It was just me and Sarah, and the friends that Grace had been staying with. A sham of a ceremony in a sad place for a tragic woman… I couldn't bear it so I left before the end.

That was when I became a real prick.*

Because I went home. I left everyone. No, not everyone, I left Tom and left Sarah and I went home. I bulk buy baked beans so that was useful. Because I was just in my bedroom. Ignoring my phone, ignoring people at the door. Sometimes with my phone off, occasionally, for a little extra flavour, with my phone on.

---

* During this I walk back until I reach the back of the wall, preferably with my face just out of the stage light.

The cotton wool feeling back, but not outside of me anymore, inside my head, a clear white fluffy fug of nothing.

A decade of sad Sunday evenings all at once, all the time.

A lot of baked beans, a lot of nothing, a lot of aborted wanks,* a lot of missed calls from my mum, a lot of missed calls from Sarah, and a lot of texts that I only saw the first three words of because I wasn't brave enough to read them.

I'm not sure exactly how long I stayed like that. (I mean I know because I've gone back and worked it out and it was two days, but at the time it could have been weeks.) Because I was just on Facebook, scrolling aimlessly through the interesting screeds of nothing to distract me from living when a picture of Tom came up, posted by a friend along with an articulate message about why they were sad he was dead.

He'd died and I hadn't been there. Just him and Sarah…

Well I hadn't liked the trailer so why should I watch the fucking film.†

Music.‡

---

* Charlie suggested this line, showing both a scary insight into my psychology and an impressive lack of taste.
† I still find this line quite difficult and don't get it right every time. I think that's because it's quite amorphous and depending on each audience and show it has to have a different combination of anger and sadness and hopelessness.
‡ This is the *ah's* falsetto joining in with 'let's die idiots together'. It makes me feel like a sad little boy. I used to cry quite a lot when I did it but that's stopped now.

I mean who can blame me, right? Except in that situation other people were having to pick up the slack that I had left. Not other people. Another person. Sarah. I suppose if I'd thought about it I would have realised I couldn't stay in my room forever but I was carefully avoiding that fact.

Then the next day, there was this van outside my window that wouldn't stop beeping its horn (that happens sometimes it's a narrow road). But it was Sarah. Standing outside the zip van leaning in through the window onto the horn and looking up my bedroom. Tired. Furious. I didn't care. I didn't care that she'd come, I didn't care that she'd got a van, I didn't care that people were leaning out of their windows shouting down at her telling her to shut up because I was in here and she was out there and there was this whole world between us but then this guy came out and he looked nasty pointing in her face, spittle-flecked. It looked like it was going to switch so I didn't have a choice, I went out wearing my ridiculous pyjamas (a Lionel Richie t-shirt and a sarong) – which incidentally will diffuse any argument – so he left and Sarah pushed me. Hard.

'How dare you James.'

Yeah. How dare I.

'I can't do this on my own, he needed us to do it together.'

There was absolutely no way –

I'd made it a lot more difficult because if I'd been around and not distracting Sarah we would have been able to get hold of Tom's body in a much more straightforward manner. However due to outstanding arrangements he'd already been taken to a chapel of rest.* Which meant we had time to plan. I had time to shower and change into my suit because I'm hilarious… and eat a final can of beans.

We arrived at seven, the place closed on the hour and Sarah introduced me to the guy in charge:

'Nigel.' Now it's important that you know that Nigel actually didn't sound anything like this but I really like doing this voice so that's what he sounds like to you. 'My name is Nigel. I work in a funeral home.'†

Sarah introduced me. 'This is James, he's very sad.'

'Now I actually close in ten minutes so chop-chop.'

They smell weird those places.

He showed us in. Tom was there, well he wasn't…his body was. Eyes sewn shut. I thought about crying thereby removing any impulse to do so. Nigel came back in:

'I'm sorry, you have to leave now. I did warn you.'

'Oh Nigel, I'm really sorry you must get this all the time but I've spent all day just trying to get James out of his house, is there any chance we could just give him five minutes on his own? I could help you close up or maybe could we have a quick cup of tea.'

---

* All of this paragraph to here is very information-giving so I got into a habit of saying it as fast as possible. This led to wondering if I could do it with the whole show which led to a speed run with Dan where I did the whole show in twenty-five minutes. I hope you are impressed. I live a very full interesting life thanks.

† All of this paragraph is done in the voice. An adenoidal nightmare.

So I had a very limited amount of time to get Tom out of there. I don't know if you've ever tried to pick up a corpse but they are heavy and they are not helping. So I managed to get him sitting up then let him fall, slowly at first, then all at once out of the coffin...and up his head on my shoulder (romantic), my hand on his arse (sexy) then waltzed him out and round the corner till we got to the security door. *

Turns out funeral homes have security doors, I don't know why – in case of Lazaruses (or Lazarai depending on what kind of an idiot you are).†

So I tried a few times waltzing fast enough but didn't work and the problem was him not helping so in the end I just sat Tom on the floor with his head against the button, went to the door and propped it with one of my shoes, went back for my buddy and danced him out... And onto the pavement where it was ridiculous because there I was standing outside a funeral home in broad daylight, cradling the corpse of my childhood friend, and a group of people were walking along the pavement straight towards us and they looked at me and they looked at him AND NONE OF THEM SAID ANYTHING. They just walked past us and went into the pub next door. I mean, what did they think I was doing? Did they think that's how people get there? Coz Tom's eyes were sewn shut and surely? It took every ounce of restraint in me not to shout after them:

---

* All of the physical 'business' (as opposed to 'pleasure' I assume) that I describe in the funeral parlour I re-create as best I can. The physical effort helps heighten the energy.

† This callback rarely works. Still do it though don't I.

'COME BACK! YOU ARE TERRIBLE CITIZENS. I'M STEALING A BODY.'

Panic contained, outrage overcome, I got Tom round the corner and laid him gently in the back of the zip van. Then ran back around picking up my shoe on the way and into the now-empty room, and closing the coffin lid just in time because as I did it Nigel and Sarah turned round the corner.

'I'm sorry. I just, couldn't look at him anymore.'

'That's okay, but why are you holding a shoe?'

'I dunno, I'm pretty messed up at the moment.'

'I understand. Sometimes you just need to hold one shoe.'*

As he turned out the lights at the front and exited onto the street with us I tried to make small talk:

'By the way Nigel, why do you have security doors?'

'Well, once there was this stag party that got in and it really wasn't amusing at – why are you interested in my security arrangements?'

Sarah interjected. 'We have to go now, James stop bothering Nigel. Thank you so much.'

'Yeah, thanks Nige.'

So we had Tom.

---

* Thank Christ for this line. It was at some point on the tour that I came up with it. Up until then the holding-a-shoe thing was something that I thought was hilarious but was rarely received that way by the audience.

I should say now that so far we had done absolutely nothing illegal. That's right people, go nuts, grab a body – not from a grave, naughty naughty, that's not allowed, but taking a corpse is not illegal because no one owns a corpse. The law empowers one or more people to take possession of a corpse for the sole purpose of disposal but 'the only lawful possessor of a corpse is the earth.' That's what it says in the Law... Books...

I read it on the *Good Funeral Guide* website but I'm pretty sure it's ironclad.

So we had Tom, what else did we need?*

A boat. And where exactly might we get a boat from?

That's right: Victoria Park, because it turns out that revenge is a dish best served fucking weird.

We waited till midnight, hopped the fence and it was actually really easy. If you ever need a boat just go to Victoria Park in east London and fill your boots. Which is all you have to do because they just tie them up out in the middle of the lake but the water's really shallow so just fill your boots.

I waded out, untied one and dragged it back to shore, over the grass, over the fence and carefully slid into the zip van next to Tom. Easy, too easy. Too easy. It was too light – the boat was made of fibreglass which is not flame-retardant. So there I was full of this realisation (it felt quite cool actually – full of soap opera emotion):

---

* I wait for the audience to answer, gathering them up in the sprint to the finish. A surprisingly large amount of hopeful people will shout out 'ship!' here.

'Sarah! It's all over! We're going to have to take him back because the boat is made of fibreglass which is *not flame-retardant!*'

'Shut up James, shut up, shut up. I'm an engineer and I told you we're going to Wickes in the morning!'

'Oh. Yeah.'

'Please promise me you will have no more ideas.'

'I promise.'

We had that feeling the whole time, where, because you're moving forward, because you're doing something, that something's all that matters. I mean there was no question or worry, just the next excellent step. We were hysterical, we couldn't sleep all night (Sarah managed to get about twenty minutes' kip at one point). The rest of the time we were just driving around. We invented a game that you can take home with you. All you need is a vehicle and a fast food drive-through. We had our van and a McDonald's. You just go round and round: 'One hamburger please... Yes it's us again!... No just the one – see you soon maybe!' Then you drive until you see someone walking home on their own and you slow right down and follow them – as soon as they notice you, you pull up alongside and roll down the window: 'Special delivery.' The rainbow of emotions that flows across a face in that scenario is truly wonderful. You don't even need a corpse in the back for it to be fun.

We turned up at Wickes the next morning, giddy and wired (which is also my stripper name – cards on the table at box office). We got what we needed: aluminium sheeting, welding kit, a big jerry can of fuel and lots of bags of kindling. Kindling because big bits of wood burn slower and cooler than little bits and we needed hot so we needed lots. We paid on credit card (grown-ups), wheeled our trolley back to the van and realised at the same time with a look of liquid terror that we had a problem. This Wickes was one where in the early morning lots of guys hang around hoping to be picked up as extra hands on building sites, so we had an audience and a stolen boat... and a corpse in the van. There was only one solution. I sat on the front seat and Sarah piled the stuff on top of me. So there we were with this audience of normal human beings:

'Mate! Mate! – You know the thing about vans is there's this whole bit behind you!'

'Aha-haa. That's not how we do a van.'

So there I was, festooned in our purchases and relieved to remember I'd packed a bottle of whisky because I can't drive so I'd designated myself drinker (and PR person of Team Viking, waving people in online) because while I'd been busy being a selfish, self-involved abortive self-abuser (or self-pleasurer – different strokes for different folks) Sarah had been busy inviting all the people who loved Tom (which was so many people) who could get to where we were going and not call the police – so only twenty or so were coming.

We'd talked about where we were going to go. I'd suggested the sea, because you know, 'Vikings,' but Sarah had pointed out, 'Tides. What did we say about ideas James?' So we decided to just go up the Thames. Sarah had found the place, not very close to anywhere and hard to get to but beautiful apparently and quiet. A bit where the Thames curved back on itself.

I remember that journey so vividly, leaving London behind as the sun rose behind us, all the colours so *bright* it's the grief superpower, that prehistoric cortex on top of our spine that spits out adrenaline when someone in our tribe dies because there might be a tiger to watch out for.

It makes everything pretty.

We turned off the A road, drove a long way down a cart track and we got there, and it was beautiful, late-morning sun dappled by a willow, stream flowing into the river, rushes swaying solemnly on the opposite bank.

Now a little advice with corpses, they're a lot like babies in that you have to support the head. Cos I'd got Tom sat up so Sarah could get the boat out past him then didn't think, had a drink, didn't care and *bfllfghfff* – that's not what it sounded like but I can't do the sound again, because I'm bad at them and it was the worst thing I've ever heard, because Tom's head had hit the bit that juts out in the back of vans and it had opened up his cheek and it turns out that they glue not sew people's eyes because it caught the corner of Tom's left eye and it peeled open trying to burst out of his head and the smell, Christ, the smell. As social media baron I requested ice, lots of ice, and Lynx Africa* (because that will cover any smell) from those due to arrive first.†

---

* Seriously though it's called *Lynx Africa*. Sometimes when I think about the colonial ramifications of that name I shudder.

† Here's a bit that I did here for ages then just forgot:
    'We carry that stuff around in us you know, when you die it's not worms that eat you first, no, they're last to the party. The lads who do the real job, the bacteria and enzymes inside us. You have them inside you right

Then Sarah got to work building the boat.

It should be clear by now that I am very much the supporting character in this story because Sarah got the welding kit out and made something pyre-proof out of a fibreglass boat. She even looked really cool as she did it, wearing sunglasses instead of goggles. As she worked I sipped slowly at my whisky, upwind of Tom, watching a magpie in the willow watching me.

People arrived with booze and music and incredulity and laughter and tears. Tim and Tara brought some fancy dress. Excellent. Tom was in his now-chilled zip van dressing room smelling like a teenage boy and we laughed and drank and screamed and danced and wept and told stories until the sun started to go down. We all filled the boat up with wood, as much as it could carry. I was in charge of the fuel (don't even bloody care mate I'll slosh the whole lot on), it soaked it up pretty easily. Sarah told me later that the fibreglass frame of the boat was a U-shape like that, and she'd put the aluminium in a V-shape to channel the flame and it can't have been welded completely shut at the bottom so the petrol…anyway. We carried Tom from van to boat accompanied by a song I'd made up the night before while Sarah had been napping. You'll recognise it.

Music.*

– now. The stuff that is going to eat us from the inside out. They'll start with the pancreas…bloody love a bit of pancreas they do.'

* I leave the song repeating over and over until I say, 'There was no music now.'

We didn't have a bow and arrow, so Sarah and I both lit matches.

It caught pretty easily and we pushed the boat out.

It drifted slowly downstream towards the sunset.

This incredible sky painted like Turner on ecstasy.

From deep red through pink and purple to lightest blue, the moon already ghosting in.

I thought back, making myself take it all in –

Flashes of memories:

Tom in his hospital, tired.

Tom on my doorstep a year ago.

Tom at Sarah's graduation accepting her degree on her behalf in character as Sarah because we'd locked her in a cupboard.

Tom waking me up on my eighteenth birthday with a bottle of champagne.

Tom punching my bully, twice his size.

Tom on the top deck of a bus tearing pages out of porn magazines and out of the window, aiming for pushchairs on the pavement below.

Tom holding on to my mum's legs, scared of the Child Catcher.

Just Tom, always Tom;

Laughing

and laughing

and laughing.

There was no music now, the only sound was the river and the snap crackle and pop of Tom drifting slowly away downstream. Standing there in the shallows I felt Sarah take my hand. I looked over to where the magpie had been and they'd been joined by a friend. Two for joy. Odin must have been happy.

'Oh Sarah, I'm so, I've been useless, I've been the worst. I'm so sorry.'

'Shut up James. It's worked out alright hasn't it?'

'Yeah, but you have to know you're a fucking wonder. You've done all of this you're incredible and all I've done is get in the way.'

'Look. I know it can't have been easy for you, caught right in the middle of all of this.'

'Yeah. Oh God, finding out he was in love with me and never said anything to us un–'

'– you mean finding out he was in love with *me* and never –'

'Bastard.'

And obviously it makes sense. He knew us, he knew exactly how to play us, the little shit. It makes sense. If he'd just asked us. He had. He knew we wouldn't do it. It makes sense. He would have been fucking delighted. It couldn't have gone better. It makes sense, it makes sense like if you pour ten litres of fuel into a boat with a nice gap for it between hull and aluminium, just like if you fill a Christmas pudding full of brandy and then set fire to it, at some point there will be repercussions. And that is when the boat exploded.

And I think that's exactly how he would have wanted to go. With his two best friends, knee deep in water, *furious.* And in two weeks' time, responsible for a seven-year-old girl finding his hand in a nearby field.

The police arrived soon after, they'd been tipped off by Nigel and traced us all the way from the CCTV cameras of McDonald's Haringey.

Sarah and I both received six month suspended sentences for a variety of offences and Sarah had her zip van account cancelled.

Here I am five years* later telling you this story,

and all of it is...†

---

* Five years is right regardless of the facts, I think because it's close enough to still feel it but far enough away that it's not too raw.

† And all of these footnotes are...
(Special shoutout to the lady on the front row in Soulby Village Hall who finished that sentence for me with a very loud, clear, 'BULLSHIT!')
If you really really *really* want to know what is true and what is not then go and look at the Appendices.

A HUNDRED DIFFERENT WORDS FOR LOVE

Set: stage right a full-size piano keyboard with a loop pedal attached.

Upstage centre an old amp with a box of matches and a sports cap water bottle on it.

I am onstage as the audience walk in.*

A preamble, talking about the venue/weather/my health/the attractiveness of the audience.

Hiya, how you doing? I'm gonna talk to you about a very rarely mentioned subject, the subject of love. Has anyone heard of it? Great. Good. Everyone else, see me after class.

This is a story about a relationship I had with a woman. Correct, not only am I white, middle-class and male, I'm also cisgender and heterosexual. I have all of the aces. There is a very good reason why this show will not receive Arts Council funding: this guy doesn't need it. Which is obviously a nice joke but actually the show I made that comes after this did get Arts Council funding which I think tells you all you need to know about the world. I have the greatest grant that nature can provide. And I used to now say – This Pigment, This Penis, This Proclivity; This Privilege...but alliteration gets laughs and it's not actually a joke. But it's interesting to mention privilege at the beginning of a show about love.

---

* I will often eat a banana or two as the audience enter. I do it before *Team Viking* as well now but the habit began during the Edinburgh run of this show. I have three reasons for doing so:

1) They are excellent for energy and I am an athlete in peak physical condition.

2) Watching someone eat a banana is funny. Especially if they know they are being watched. I urge you to use this in your everyday life.

3) Bananas are delicious.

You know the pyramid thing – Maslow's Hierarchy of Needs? At the bottom, there's food for eating, air for breathing, love doesn't come into it till halfway up and storytelling shows don't even register on the pyramid, which I imagine is an oversight... Love is a privilege. And I don't know what this is for. That being said I hope that I justify your attendance by touching you...on a level that merits it.*

I wonder if it'll be one of those shows where he says the title in the show?

Now, I'll go and do the lights and when I come back I'll be a performer and all the rest of this will be artifice.†

Hello, my name is James, I'm going to tell you a story and none of it is true.‡

I call upon Aphrodite (with a bit of help from Ludus) to aid me in this account.§

***

Music.¶

I stand: leg shaking, impatiently waiting for the tube doors.

---

* I've sort of done footnotes in the actual show here. That's how much I like them. 'Touching you' is always directed at the closest man in the audience.

† HOLY CRAP HE'S DONE IT AGAIN

‡ SORRY FOR BLOWING YOUR MIND

§ Before anyone says anything about mixing pantheons, hold off. I got this.

¶ All of the writing in the indented sections is spoken over piano music on the loop pedal. The chord structure is C/Am/F/Dm until further notice. That particular progression has an unfinished sound to it.

It's Saturday morning and I'm really quite late.

The doors slide open and I slip through, zone two, platform empty, just me, no wait: one, two, three tube mice getting on with another day in paradise.

I'd love to stay but I can't delay, I'd run but I wouldn't make it all the way, so fast walking is the order of the day.

Up the stairs, through the barriers and out, blinded by the sun; laser scowling, autumn sharp into my eyes as I turn the corner, clenched bum quick strides.

I fish the keys out, up two floors and in, straight to the freezer, where I squeeze out all ten Viennettas (still in Sainsbury's bags).*

Then I realise there is really no reason for me to rush because I've not booked a taxi yet.

Phone out, a text from Giles. 'Are you on time?' No Giles. No I'm not. Call a cab…fifteen minutes…perfect, why should it be sooner?

I sit down. I stand back up. I put the Viennettas back in the freezer (I'm not an idiot).†

I lean against the fridge and look out on a familiar room: dangerously transparent glass table, terrible carpet. The sofa.

---

* People always laugh when I say Viennettas which just goes to show what a dangerous tool nostalgia could be in the hands of a sociopathic writer or performer. Thankfully no writers or performers are sociopaths.

† I *am* an idiot.

I slowly sink down to freezer-level and from there I remember the last time I looked at this room from this recumbent position.

***

It was three years ago, three in the morning. Sarah, my best friend, brilliant, hilarious, engineer, has got engaged to Emma and so we are having a party.* There had been grown-ups earlier (Emma's parents, not Sarah's dad Giles) but they'd left and I'd suggested that only one of Sarah's infamous house parties could be the proper way of finishing off the occasion. The music choices have degenerated, the soundtrack now oscillating wildly between Disney hits and 90s bangers depending which league of dangerous idiots had control of Spotify, and no one is drinking recognisable things anymore, it's now like: 'Absinthe and ginger beer? Perfect I'll have two pints.' A shit glitter ball lights the scene. And I'm sat with my head against the frosted-over freezer. There's limited ice left at the party so it was my only choice for preventing a severe concussion. Emma's sitting next to me – it's very much her fault I'm here. A short bit of advice about replicating the famous *Dirty Dancing* lift when you are drunk at a party: don't.

And she walks up to me...

I'm not going to tell you her name by the way, I've thought about it and I don't want to. I'm not going to tell you her name or what she looks like or anything about her. So when I'm being her in this story I'm going to look a lot like me and sound

---

* I'm still not sure about this line. I think I'm gonna try and fix it on tour because it's just boring isn't it.

like me too but hopefully you'll know who's who because of the powerful acting, don't worry though you will get some characterisation, I play two older people and an American (I'm famous for my accent work). So: money's worth.

But actually could you all just close your eyes for a minute, just for a minute, now imagine her. Imagine this woman. Imagine what she looks like...and imagine her a name. Thank you, you can open your eyes. In this story she's the Girl* because I'm the Boy.

And she comes up to me, walks over from where they're dancing and comes straight towards me. I've seen her before, other places, other times, other parties. She knows Sarah – I'm not sure how but out of nowhere she decides to walk towards me and I'm looking at her and I'm ready, I'm looking at her and she's looking at...

The fridge above my head, and she opens the door, the light shines on her face, now that's the only thing I want to look at, she takes out a bottle of wine, tops up her glass, and is about to walk out of my life so I say:

'Hi!'

She looks down.

---

* I hope that people forgive my use of the word 'Girl' here because of the context. I have often considered changing it to 'Woman'† but something about that doesn't quite work. I use 'Girl' because the show is about a young love and reluctantly because of Richard Curtis. This show has a tricky relationship with that man and his movies.

† Although 'The Woman' would be a lovely reference to Sherlock Holmes.

'Hello. That's a normal thing to be doing. Are you alright?'

'Yeah, yeah. I'm just an incredibly dirty dancer.'

She laughs.

Emma interjects: 'Do you two know each other?'

'Yeah, yeah, yeah this is…' (She says her name.) 'We go way back.' (We'd never talked before.) We talk, Emma leaves when it's clear that we're not desperate to have her input into our conversation (she winks at me as she goes which I find rude, patronising, I don't know why you'd wink at me, I'm just having a pleasant chat with an interesting stranger). I manage to leave the freezer; she gave me the courage to leave the freezer because I just wanted to keep talking to her. We stand by the window, I smoke cigarettes, she might have had one, I don't remember. She seems…nice. Turns out she lives with Simon, Sarah's colleague. They get a taxi home.

Last person standing, me, obviously. Sarah had fallen asleep on the floor so Emma and I carried her to bed. SHE IS HEAVIER THAN SHE LOOKS. Dense. Like a dark star, galaxies in each one of her limbs,* we put her to bed and I staggered to the cupboard, pulled the quilt out and made it over to the sofa where I fell unconscious face down with my trousers and pants inexplicably around my ankles and I like to imagine a happy smile on my face.

---

* The eagle-brained reader may not have guessed but the character of Sarah is based partly on my friend Charlie Covell otherwise known as 'The Fat-Ankled Foot Soldier of Satan'.

Two weeks later and I'm at work. A promo job for Chick Fillet; an American chicken sandwich restaurant.* I am to be their mascot, a massive cow, black and white, no genitals (definitely no bull) and holding a sign that reads: *Eat More Chicken.* The guy in charge had been very clear about my role:

I affect a TERRIBLE American accent.

'Yeah, so. It's really simple. Two rules. The cow doesn't speak he never speaks. No sounds at all, no human sounds no cow sounds.'

'Right, sure.'

'And you're soft so people are gonna wanna hug you but you can't let them; you can't touch anyone, you can't touch the kiddies.'

'Is there any other way you can put that?'

'You can't touch the kiddies.'

---

* I cut all of these bits to keep the story moving: 'They decided to do a test day over here, dipping their toe into the ocean of fried chicken that is London (I've since discovered, Chick Fillet donated a lot of money to Trump, anti-abortion, very right wing, you can never be certain but I think they're the bad guys). That's by the by, I was dressed as a big cow. That's their mascot. A pretty good metaphor for meat-eating as establishment politics, just getting the underclasses to fight amongst themselves.'
'They'd taken over an Argentinian Steak restaurant. Steak. I looked like a protest. Another level of irony. You couldn't make it up.'
I'm gonna put in a few bits that I cut. This is not as my friend Camilla suggested to 'up my word count'. Not least because footnotes don't count towards a word count.† I'm doing it to give you a sense of how the shows get made.

† Which I'm absolutely fine with by the way. Happy if anything.

'Oh there isn't.'

So I'm standing on the street corner. Holding this sign.* I'd
smuggled my headphones in with me, and I'd made myself
a classical *moosic* playlist: Beethoven's 'Pastoral Symphony',
Saint-Saëns' 'The Carnival of the Animals' and 'The Bad
Touch' by the Bloodhound Gang.† There I am, ruminating
in my own happy haze, chewing the cud. When suddenly
out of the anonymous pedestrians, some twenty yards away
appeared the girl. The one from the party. And she's walking
down the pavement straight towards me and she's smiling so
I don't think, I just lurch towards her as if I've been pulled by
bungee... But when I get to her she turns away and stands
waiting at the traffic lights – because of course she hadn't been
walking to you James, she was just looking at the only cow
on the pavement on her way to cross the road – so I try and
style-act all cow-casual and spin on my heel but I'm much
wider than I'm used to so I just smash her in the back of the
head with the sign. Then run away.

'Seriously!? You big milky bastard! Come back!'

I turn back. Mortified but masked by the twin cloaks of
massive mammal and silence.

And it's adorable because I'm looking straight at her face
through the mesh in the neck and she's looking at the cow's
eyes some two feet above her own.

---

* I did this job. I did not fall in love as a result. I ate my body weight in
chicken burgers and felt ill.
† Cultured *and* hilarious? Incidentally I would never make this playlist. I
don't like Saint-Saëns.

'Did, did you just hit me?!'

Slow sad nod.

'Why did you do that?'

Complicated sign language.

'Are you not allowed to speak?'

Shake head, nod head, shake head, confused wobble.

'Alright Daisy, give me a hug.'

Sigh and slump. *

At this point I should say that I am very much the child of Richard Curtis... Ah I know how that sounds. I am not *the* child of Richard Curtis, I am *a* child of Richard Curtis (if I was the child of Richard Curtis none of this would be happening, I'd be in Hollywood).†

I grew up swaddled in the example of binary monogamous heterosexual relationships and few of my examples differed

---

* This scene is AHDWFL's equivalent of the Nigel/shoe scene. I *know* it is funnier than I'm making it but I haven't quite worked it out yet. Only done the show thirty times.

† Literally no idea why so many reviewers talked about Richard Curtis. Sure, the show is partly written as a deliberate undermining of Richard Curtis' stupid saccharine legacy but there's more to it than that so why does everyone always go on about Richard Curtis?

I tried adding a bit that went: 'I mean I don't *like* Richard Curtis but it's family isn't it? You don't have to like them.' But I think it appeared as if I was just saying Richard Curtis again. Richard Curtis. Richard Curtis.

Richard Curtis.

I'm fine.

from those prevailing socio-cultural norms. Then as an adolescent when I was looking for new examples to follow, it was *Four Weddings*, *Notting Hill* and their innumerable offspring that took over my teaching. So somewhere deep down inside me is this deeply inculcated thing, that despite my rationally knowing that it's not real, it's not true, we don't live in a binary universe, we are free inside ourselves to be whoever we want and love whoever we love, part of me, beneath that understanding, thinks that it is, that I do, that I don't, that I won't, that I can't. Which is shit…

But it's not all bad because I think it would be impossible to be influenced by that quixotic and yet restrained romantic heritage and then look a gift cow in the mouth.

So I called Sarah straight away.

'Mate, the girl who lives with Simon – they're not together are they?'

'Hello James nice to hear from you I'm well, thanks for asking. No they're not, is there anything else I can do for you?'

'No thank you. I'll explain later.'

I got Sarah and Simon, the SS, to –

I got Sarah AND Simon, the SAS (who dares wins), to sort –

I didn't care if it was Sarah OR Simon, it was an SOS, a cry for help.* I just wanted to see the Girl again.

I'll spare you the details of the dinner party, more for my sake than yours. It finishes like this: I am face down on the

---

* This was very much Daniel's idea. Both he and I bloody love a pun.

terrible carpet really banging my head on the floor. Because I'd been terrible. I'd been the worst: I'd purported to hold some views that I really don't just in order to have a stake in the conversation. I think I barked like a dog instead of laughing at one point? I'd been aware of every awkward pore of my skin. And Sarah and Emma are sitting on the sofa clinically dissecting my disastrous performance like *Match of the Day* pundits. Cutting off this brutal anatomising[*] Emma nudged Sarah:

'Go on, you should tell him.'

Sarah sighed. 'The thing is James you were terrible, but she gave me her phone number for you if you want it.'

So I played it super cool. I texted her immediately:

It was really nice to see you would you like to go for a drink sometime?

She did not respond.

For forty minutes. Fo-o-o-rty minutes. I died a thousand times in those forty minutes, eventually though – beep beep – who's this, someone from my past?

It was nice to see you too. Yes a drink sometime would be nice.

Two 'nice's[†], no kiss, I'll take it though. So she's waited for forty minutes so I waited forty seconds. I texted her immediately:

How about tomorrow night? I'm free tomorrow night, would you like a drink tomorrow night?

---

[*]   'Brutal anatomising' was 'excruciating post-match analysis' until I did the show in the Anatomy Lecture Theatre in Summerhall.
[†]   That word 'nice' again.

Which I think we can all agree is a text that only *Macbeth* would send.* Somehow though, she refrained from burning down her house, putting on a false moustache and purchasing plane tickets to Panama, she actually replied:

Not free 'tomorrow night'. (Quotation marks, hilarious.) *How about Friday?*

I replied:

AFFIRMATIVE

Before I could ruin it any further.†

I was not free on the Friday…but my nieces will forgive me. My sister won't, but my nieces will. I had to say I was free because if I hadn't said yes, if I'd said I was busy on Friday then who knows? We keep on trying to get a date in the diary, we keep on missing each other and then three months later we bump into each other on a street corner and she's pregnant with someone else's baby and I'm alone for the rest of my life. So I said I was free.

It was Friday the 27th of October, does that mean anything to anyone?‡ No? But it's close to something isn't it, what's it close to?

---

* This line is better than the one I was doing before. 'At least there could be no confusion about when I was mooting a meeting' – no matter how satisfying 'mooting a meeting' is to say.

† This whole exchange get lots of laughs of recognition and much like the porn/hedges bit in *Team Viking*, I'm sure that it's well-worn comic territory. I'm cheap. I'm also legitimately terrible at messaging.

‡ I often get people saying that it is close to, or their birthday. Which I thought was weird but then someone explained the maths to me. My favourite was a woman shouting, 'Oh yes!' and when I said 'Oh?' she said 'No, I was thinking of February.'

Halloween, exactly. So our walk down the South Bank was going to be different than I'd expected. (I thought a walk down through a nice bit of London, you're not concentrating on something else like a film or a play, you don't have to look at each other all the time and most importantly you are not in a bar on a Friday night in London which is nightmarish even without the holiday costume choices.) We met at Westminster. (As my niece would say, 'next to a church called Abby'.) I thought that she'd stood me up for a while but eventually she arrived. We crossed the bridge; the only humans in a sea of zombies, vampires and corpses. Turned along the South Bank through the magical fairy lights, past the magical invisible homeless people. She's walking quite close to me, her arm brushing against mine, which is exciting. We stop off to get a coffee at the National, continue our walk.* She talks about her family, I talk about my friends. She seems nice.

We get to London Bridge and she has to go – she has work early the next morning. We're standing at the top of the stairs to the underground and she's right here, this close: kissing distance.

I know it was kissing distance because I've checked, I've had stone-cold verification from a victim. I just for some reason,

---

* 'When we come out there's a busker, a one-man band, his song starts with guitar or whatever and there's a rhythm to it, then the vocals come in and then the kick pedal starts and that's the heartbeat, because the song's been missing something till it's there. Bm-bm-bm-bm and you know that at some point the pedal is going to miss a beat and that's when the song'll get to the good bit...' This was a plant for a later callback, I'll tell you when we get there.

like, I think my eyes are fine, I just don't recognise kissing distance.*

I said: 'This has been nice, we should do it again sometime.' (Which I was pleased with, astonished in fact at my audacity in not adding a modifying 'maybe' to protect myself.)

And she responds but I can't hear her because the million wriggling creatures in my stomach are shutting down my brain. So like a legend I repeat myself:

'This has been nice, we should do it again sometime.'

She laughs

and she gives me a kiss. Just here.

So mainly beard, but I'll take it.

And she walks down the stairs and as she walks down the stairs I realise.

I realise.

I realise that that's the way I go home. Like, I go home that way, but I can't go that way now, I can't be like:

'Haha. I'm not following you, I'm not following you.'

Because it seems like you are definitely following them.

So all I could do is stand outside London Bridge for five minutes like a lemon that looks exactly like me. Eventually, that seems like enough and I –

---

* I feel quite a lot more exposed with the shows being written down than I do performing them. I can't distract you by prancing around. Wait. Is that why I've done footnotes? Holy crap.

and she's walking back up the stairs towards me – we both freeze like the other one is a T-Rex that only responds to movement. Eventually she breaks the impasse:

'That's not the way I go home, I don't go home that way, I get the bus from over there but we said goodbye and we weren't moving so I panicked and went down the stairs. Why are you still here?'

I was like, 'That is the way that I go home, I go home that way. I'm not following you –'

She's walking up the stairs towards me, she's walking up, she's right here.

'Okay. Bye.'

And that is the end of story number one.* We never saw each other again.

Nah, we got together; despite our mutual shit-ness we somehow managed to make it work. Which was good.

It was really good.

***

Music.

Now the taxi's at the door, I've got the Viennettas back out of the freezer, and I'm running down the stairs taking them three at a time – two at a time actually three at a time is quite dangerous – into the back of the car:

---

* I mean. How many nascent romances have been nipped in the bud because of a lack of forthrightness. It's lots right? I'm telling myself it's lots.

'Is it James?' (I know it sounds stereotypical but this taxi driver really was from Cockney land.)

'Yeah, I'm really sorry but I'm running quite late, is there any chance you can go as fast as possible.'

'Mate you just literally described my job to me: my job is to take you where you are going as fast as possible.'

'I know I'm sorry, I'm really sorry, it's just the person I'm picking up is quite elderly and I've got all these Viennettas here.'

'Viennettas? You should have said.'

I'm mean he's joking but that's the point when the traffic opens up and he really does step on it.

***

Three months in; three months after we got together, and we've gone to stay with her parents in the Lake District. We arrived late on Friday night so they didn't disturb us Saturday morning. From under the covers, light streaming through the window, we hear them get up, have breakfast and leave the cottage for a walk. Dozing and holding each other as their voices diminuendo down the hill replaced by birdsong.

I go to make tea, naughtily naked in an unfamiliar kitchen. Do the deed, take them back in...

there she is. Just her face sticking out.

'That kitchen is so good. Everything's in the right place, the tea bags above the kettle, the sink right next to the bin.* It's perfect. It's like you.'

'James. Are you calling me a kitchen?'

'Yes. That's exactly what I'm doing, that's how metaphors work. You are the perfect kitchen. In fact you're too perfect. So perfect that I'm going to have to kill you.' I pick up a pillow and begin to stifle her,† she fights back and we wrestle: sheets flying, laughing, kissing, tickling, our own red-cheeked romantic cliché. She ends up on top of me (she's very strong), looking down.

'James, I love you.'

One.

That wasn't our first weekend away. Our first weeken– well the day after our walk along the South Bank, I got a phone call, very early.

'Hello?'

'Hi, it's me, I had a really nice time yesterday.'

'Me too. Is everything alright?'

'Yes look just found out I've won a weekend away at Center Parcs next week and I thought I'd ask my friends but then

---

* I cannot be clear enough on this. If your tea bags are not next to your kettle then you need to address that immediately.

† Right. So far we've ticked off *Romeo and Juliet*, *Macbeth* and here we have *Othello*. Can you spot *Hamlet* and *King Lear*? (As of the 15th of March I'd rather die of poisoning from a snakebite than count *Julius Caesar* or *Anthony & Cleopatra* as tragedies.)

I thought I'd ask you first, obviously if you say yes I won't invite my friends, that'd be weird, I mean it will be weird, it's Center Parcs it'll definitely be weird, this is weird, what I'm doing now is weird isn't it? Anyway. What do you think?'

'Yes. I think yes. Please. Thank you.'

She drove. I remember our first walk there, just feeling giddy, high, my arms swinging until they snagged, caught and she held me in her hand like I was a helium balloon. It was a wonderful weekend. Went swimming, ate terrible food, did laser clay pigeon shooting (don't bother). We mainly stayed in the chalet though. It was amazing.*

Sheets flying, laughing, kissing, tickling, our own red-cheeked romantic cliché. She ends up on top of me (she's very strong), looking down.

'James, I love you.'

One.

Two.

Six weeks in, six weeks after we got together and we had our first argument. Sunday, we were having breakfast, two in the afternoon, the flat to ourselves, wrapped in sheets and hypothesising about potential beautiful futures together and I can't remember exactly when it started but it was around the time I said:

---

* This is where the callback to the busker used to sit: 'The drum skipped a beat, the song got to the good bit.' Which is theft from my favourite romantic story of all time, Fenny and Arthur in Douglas Adams' *So Long, and Thanks for all the Fish*. It sounded a bit smug though.

'I don't want to get married, not ever, I think it's stupid.'

And she said something about me assuming things about her opinions and so I just explained it to her; all my thoroughly thought-through reasons for rejecting the institution. And that seemed to make her more angry, so I just started from the beginning again but slower this time and using smaller words…and for some reason it just degenerated from there. It was just me and then her then me and then her and then me and then her – both of us furious at the lack of tessellation between us – me and then her and then me and then her and then me until –

'YOU KNOW THE SUN IS JUST A STAR, JAMES!'

'I'm sorry what?'

'The sun is just a star.'

Now that's a fairly straightforward metaphor for perspective but by this point in the argument I thought the rules of engagement in this bar fight were that we leave the guns of articulacy at the door. So there I was, reeling from this…

'Where, where did that come from?'

'You know the sun is just a star.'

I apologised. She forgave me. We moved on.

– our own red-cheeked romantic cliché. She ends up on top of me (she's very strong), looking down.

'James, I love you.'

One.

Two.

Three.*

I said 'I love you.'

To Sarah. Six months in, six months after we got together, and we went away for a weekend in Brighton; Sarah, Emma, the girl and I. Ostensibly to help them plan their wedding. They were on the brink of putting down a deposit on the venue. We only just made our train, the girl (delayed by something) diving through the train doors as they beeped closed. We dumped our bags and went for a walk, they were all laughing about what I would be wearing. Then Sarah got a call from her dad, Giles. He is a difficult man, he didn't speak to Sarah for two years after she came out. They only started talking again when her mum died. Breast cancer. So she hadn't told him about the engagement but he must have asked what she was doing because she simply replied:

'Planning my wedding to Emma, Dad, we're getting married.'

And I didn't hear the rest of the conversation but it wasn't good. Neither was the one after, back at the Airbnb. So sad, so angry. Emma suggested the only thing she could, that they postpone the wedding, just delay until it could happen without this rich seam of grief running through the middle of it. It was too much, so sad, so angry, 'Fuck him, fuck you for even suggesting that, no, NO we can't let him ruin this like

---

* The magic number. Ah, it always bothers me to reinforce accepted wisdom but it's just a thing. Three works. Threes work. It's nice that here, directly in the middle of a cycle of three shows where I use sequences of three quite a lot, I'm bellowing the number three out at the audience. Subtle.

he's ruined everything else.' It was too heated too much, so Emma went out for a walk, I had nothing, helpless in the face of my friend's pain. The girl was incredible, she just listened to Sarah, listened her down. All I could offer was a hug. Just trying to squeeze her okay.

'I love you.'*

I saw a flicker on the girl's face over Sarah's shoulder.

Looking down.†

'James, I love you.'

One.

Two.

Three.

Four.

Four seconds is too long.

She gets up off me and goes for a shower without looking back.‡

The Ancient Greeks had six words for love, didn't they? Does anyone know them? Eros – sexy times; Agape – love for

---

* When making the show, Daniel really created this whole act. He suggested the structure and also most of the matter. The three occasions seem very natural and obvious now but it took ages to settle on what they were. Look at that structure though. Dan Goldman, what a guy.
† I do a mime of 'she's very strong'.
‡ I always act this out and from the back corner of the stage. Stop and take a minute. Then go to get my water and do the next section with water bottle.

everyone; Philia – love for your friends; Pragma – pragmatic love; Philautia – nobody knows, lost to history (self love), and Ludus – playful love. Six words. Six words isn't enough.*

So what about Eskimos? (Or Inuits, *Yu pik.*) They have fifty different words for snow right?† And living where they do, they feel it in their fingers, they feel it in their toes, snow really is all around them and so their vocab grows. But I think even Eskimos would agree that love is a more multifaceted concept than snow. So more than six, more than fifty. Say *a hundred...*‡

Like all of us here, we've probably all used the word love at least once today already, possibly something that you've forgotten, possibly about something that you don't even like maybe BUT you said that you *love* it§ and at the same time as it being that base utility word we also expect and hope it to be the most important word you will ever say to anyone.

And that was the point, because I'd said it to someone before and I'd meant it (I know, that's why they call me Ol' Jimmy

---

* Okay saddle up. The Greeks did not have six words for love. Sorry. For a start, Ludus is Roman. Sorry to everyone I have lied to. In my defence I was thoroughly misled by the School of Life, a philosophy school in Bloomsbury ran by Alain De Botton. (Pretentious toi?) It could be that there are four words but now I don't know who to trust. I know it's not Alain De Botton, fuck that guy.

† Again, this may rattle a feather or ruffle a cage but it is absolutely true. It may seem entirely hypocritical to glibly brag about the lies I tell about the Greek words and now be a stickler for the facts when it comes to this but, well, I'm a hypocrite. Also the word Eskimo *is* offensive but only if you are talking about the Inuit or Yupik people in Canada or Greenland, elsewhere it's totally fine.

‡ I imply the title of the show, calling back to the beginning.

§ In Edinburgh I added: 'I mean this is the Edinburgh Festival I'm sure that all of us very earnestly have said, "I would *love* to see your show."'

two girlfriends) and I'd been everywhere with her. Every park, every bar, every place, all of my friends had met that ex-girlfriend.

The whole of my life a palimpsest:* a picture painted over and over, a paper reused by a scribe, every park, every bar and every word had been written on already. My canvas thick with memories.†

So I couldn't say, 'I love you.'

But that didn't matter because I loved her, because we shared so many intimates together. I think when you share an intimacy with a person it's like you're taking a needle and thread, and just looping that emotional cotton between you. Through your skin and linking you to each other, it might be one or two, they might be innumerable, but building up and over and in and out and around until you are knit together…

And it's those feelings that count, right? Rather than the words you use to describe them, because all words are just vessels or vehicles for meaning. Words are just approximate metaphors for feelings, and you can be more specific with a collection of words, with a whole real metaphor. Like batteries, because we all carry batteries with us and they come with this image of them on computers and phones of being empty or full or a certain percentage but that's not how they work, their mass doesn't change, you can't count a charge in a percentage – no one actually knows how batteries work. It's that the image is a

---

* This incredibly apposite and beautiful analogy is brought to you by Daniel Goldman.

† I have put the water bottle down by now, if you were worried.

more useful way of us getting on… Maybe metaphors would be better: a hundred different metaphors for love. Perhaps that should be the title of the show.

I couldn't say I love you.*

Not then. Not ever. And I explained myself, tried to explain all of that and she understood. She didn't love it but she understood. And I think that's one of the fundamentals you have to have to qualify as a real relationship. Forgiving the flaws.†

***

Music.

We pull up outside Euston Station. Not outside. 'Nobody can park directly outside.' So we're round the corner. I'm out, down the pavement and in, onto the concourse…where is she…where is she. There she is, little old lady sitting down looking grumpy.

'I'm so sorry I'm so late, I'm really sorry, but we've got to run though.'

---

* What is at stake here is my ability to ever be able to commit to words. It's just seen through the lens of a relationship because they are more important.

† I worry that because I do not talk about the Girl in any detail at all that it comes across as if I'm implying here that in our relationship it fell upon the woman to forgive the failings of the man BUT this point leads on to a wider thing. I spend so much time in all three of the shows displaying my perceptions of my faults in a safe fashion that perhaps what I am actually doing is excusing them. Self-defining as a dickhead is no excuse for behaving like a dickhead. This footnote itself is getting into Russian doll-style examples of this sort of shit.

'James! I'm eighty-seven years old and my hips are one and three respectively, I literally *cannot* run,' she bursts into a massive peal of laughter and gives me a hug right around my waist (she really is that small).

'Come on you, you can carry my bag.' As we wander out she links her arm in mine. 'I thought you'd be wearing…?'

'It's in the taxi, I'll change when we get there.'

I put her bag into the boot as she slides onto the back seat and instantly becomes best friends with the cab driver. An incredible woman, Sarah's nan.[*]

It's actually down to Sarah's nan that the wedding is happening at all because when she found out the reason for the wedding being postponed she made it her life's goal to remove that impediment: her son Giles. Now obviously this took months, it took more than a year, but because this is a show I'm going to boil it down to an exchange of three lines:

'Giles! It's her life not yours and you have to let her live it.'

'Well, I just don't understand why they have to call it marriage and if she's old enough to make these sorts of decisions she's certainly old enough to listen to her father's opinions.'

---

[*] Sarah's nan is the best person. I'm not quite sure where the characterisation came from but I think a young ish man doing an impression of a forthright old lady will seem Pythonesque. I hope that her being brilliant avoids that; she certainly seems to get laughs at the right places.

'Your opinions Giles, well, what's your opinion on this: if it had been an option when I'd been a gal you'd probably never have been born. You have to celebrate change Giles.'

***

We broke up.[*]

Two years in, two years after we got together. We started breaking up. All those threads started pulling out one by one and there were so many of them.

I'm aware that's quite a leap time-wise, I'm eliding eighteen months, the most happy, the most – and I think I know why, two reasons. First, because it's sad, it's painful, and second because it's hard to contain contentment with words... So I've been doing a thing, every show I take a match and while it's lit I try to explain afresh what it was like.

I light a match and try and find the words but there are none.[†]

Sometimes it doesn't work.

I will say this: there's no joy like making someone you love happy, is there.[‡]

I can tell you why we didn't break up, because we talked a lot about it. There were some things that happened while we were together that could have been reasons for a break-up.

---

[*] I try and say this on the half-volley so it is jarring.

[†] This bit is difficult. Sometimes because it's sad, sometimes because I feel like I'm not really there, not really doing the thing I say I'm doing.

[‡] I once thought of the perfect supplementary line to go with this and I forgot it before I wrote it down.

We didn't break up because her stepdad died. He was run over by a fire engine which was horrible, sudden, hard for her and her family, I felt quite excluded from the grief at the same time as just wanting to be there for her. He was a lovely man.

We didn't break up because we argued. Which we did a lot, half for fun half not. About stupid things, like her absolute cast-iron resolve to never, ever watch a *Star Wars* film.*

It wasn't because I was sad although I was sad, I didn't realise properly at the time but I was quite sad. That's the way it works sometimes I guess. I thought I was happy because my life with her was happy and because my life with friends was happy but looking back... I was sad as well.

Those are just some of the things that can happen when you're with someone, they happened while we were together. None of them are the reason why we broke up.

It just didn't work anymore.

I pick up the water bottle and have a few sips.†

If I can put it down to anything, it could have been the fact that I hadn't set my sights on any sort of a future for us or any kind of a future at all. I'm a very mindful person (buzzword). I have so much fun enjoying the present that I neglect to think

---

* 'It wasn't because she was sexually assaulted, which she was while we were together. A man grabbed her at a bar, touched her and kissed her, someone she worked with. That was difficult. I reacted badly. My first reaction was jealousy. Not for long but that was my first reaction. I don't say that to self-flagellate, I just think it's important to register that you can always be a dick and always try harder not to be.' This used to be in this bit. I changed it because I don't think it was helping, well, anything.

† Why on earth would I mention that?

about the future. So future James really hates past James, because past James doesn't give a shit about that guy, it's like:

*I pour all of the water slowly over my head.**

Because this is great. I feel like I'm in a music video. I'm enjoying your laughter. It's great. This is great. It's hard to stop enjoying it while you're still laughing.

Water bottle empties.

But let's wait.

So there's that. There's also the thing that – it's not for me to take ownership of but I am going to talk about it. Children. Babies. Big boys and girls stuff. Because despite the fact that the world is overpopulated, our culture projects that wanting to procreate is a prerequisite to being a proper person. And I understand that we have had this hard-wired and come from thousands of years of successful shaggers but surely being evolved is being able to overcome those evolutionary imperatives that we don't need anymore.

That's the world though, what about us?

Well, I can probably have kids until the day I die but if you're a woman, if you're the girl, you can't.

Which is unfair because I can change my mind.

And it certainly didn't help. It certainly, possibly, doesn't help.

---

* There we are. I considered at this point having a pint glass that I slowly edged off a table until it smashed on the floor as if I was a horrible, hilarious cat. This all seemed like too much effort though, which is how I ended up with the water. Which is much better thematically and visually. Once more laziness coming to my aid.

It certainly, possibly, definitely, maybe doesn't help when someone in a relationship isn't thinking about the future at all.

We broke up, all those threads came out one by one, ripped, pulling the skin with them, nerves open to the world. The positive current from the battery of our love switched to the negative, not our happiness making each other happy, our sadness making each other sadder. She let go of me and I drifted up, up, up above my life, watching this stranger James carry on.* It lasted ages, way longer than it should have done because neither of us could bear to finish it, but trying to make it work was like trying to stick a leaf back on a tree...

The whole time I didn't cry. I couldn't. My heart drowning in the tears I couldn't shed.

***

Music.

We pull up outside the venue, I grab the Viennettas and dash out.

'I'm really sorry, I've got to get these to the caterers.'

'Don't worry about it James, I'll pay for the taxi, you cheap git.'

Sarah and Emma have decided they can do what they want so everyone is having Viennettas at their wedding. I hand the ice cream over to the kitchen and

---

*   All of the metaphors from early being inverted here. I tried to put as many pairs in AHDWFL as possible despite the obvious necessary fidelity to the rule of three, it changes the way things feel and is absolutely less satisfying for everyone.

head straight to the gents' toilet where I get changed into my dress.* I'm wearing a dress for the wedding. Sarah and I and our childhood friend Tom had made an agreement that when we got married we'd all be 'best men of honour' for each other and Tom and I added the proviso that we all had to wear dresses because Sarah hates wearing dresses. Obviously Tom and I were stacking the odds in our favour like nascent bookies because women couldn't marry women. Times change though and it's good to celebrate that. Talk about silver linings. Unbelievable. Our friend Tom died when he was twenty-five, I've told a story about it before. So I have to wear a dress for him as well as for Sarah. I check myself in the mirror, slip my shoes on and head out looking for compliments. I poke my head out of the door and see Giles who smiles, but as I emerge he blanches and walks past me as if we've never met before in our lives. I am mollified however by Sarah's nan who wolf-whistles and gives me a round of applause. Nearly everyone's here... No sign of the Girl yet. Obviously the girl is invited. She'll be there. Sarah asked if I wanted her not to come but that would have been ridiculous. Ceremony starting soon.

***

Three different sorts of things that got me through the sad times, the worst times and – I don't want to overwhelm you with sesquipadelia, I'm aware I hide my fragile emotional

---

* I have a lovely dress. I get changed as I talk here and hand my diverted clothes to men in the audience for them to hold. I try to be done by the time it says so in the speech.

masculinity behind a veneer of intellectual articulacy. I am, as Emma describes me, a bit of a 'wordy cunt'* but bear with me. I'll call them big things, medium things and little things. Make space in the old head box for these lofty concepts:

The big things. Friendship. Sarah was incredible, so was Emma. I spent a lot of time on the sofa. I now feel more at home on that sofa than I do in any bed I've ever slept in.

Medium things: I needed to do something to fill the void so I started to work quite hard and being busy was really good, really useful. I know that when times are hard it's not always possible to work but it was good for me.

And little things, little things all the time everywhere,† too many to numerate, but I'll tell you my favourite which is tube

---

* This particular appellation is yours courtesy of Paul Flannery: comedian and vagabond. Paul makes the show *Knightmare Live!,* which I do and is responsible for keeping me sane by giving me the chance to perform with my best friends. Doing the *Songs of Friendship* is immensely rewarding but it can be fairly isolating. In fact, today, I'm at home writing this instead of going to play a stupid made-up sport called Volfsball (worth a Google) then eating a lovely meal (Paul is an incredible cook as well as musician, entrepreneur and marijuana smoker) and playing excellent board games. Sacrifice, for your pleasure. ENJOY THIS OR I COULD HAVE BEEN THERE.

† 'Mainly tube-related from me, there are loads, so many, but I'll tell you my top three.

I was on my way somewhere. Alone, the abyss inside overwhelming. Busy, I'd made some life mistakes because I was on the tube at rush hour, and there was a baby that was so happy to be on the tube gazing up around alert at everyone's faces and just laughing with joyful wonder of being so close to so many people. It was infectious to the extent that the whole carriage was laughing with it after a couple of stops...new people cramming on confused by the communal delight.

Another time, I was going around a corner, there was a train leaving, I was in no rush, and someone barged past me, really jolted me, to get past in time. Don't do that, that's rude, there will be another one in two minutes.

mice because they're the best. I think we can all agree that they live in the shittest house in the world and they're still having a great time. They can't hear because the trains are so loud so they have to do everything through vibrations but they're still having a great time. 'Guys, guys! I found another McDonald's!* It's party time!' They are dirty, they are deaf and they are undefeated and if they can live their life and not be self-indulgent then why can't I?

Also, helping plan the wedding was good as well, well...not that terrible.

***

Music.†

And now it's time, we're all invited up the stairs and ushered into a room that looks like an enthusiastic carpenter's re-imagining of a Greek amphitheatre‡. Giles on the front row, louring over the occasion, Sarah's nan next to him keeping an eye on him.

So I was furious as I saw her sprinting towards the doors when she dropped her phone! Ha! That's what you get for being a prick. The doors started to beep and close as she leant down to pick up the phone and then executed a perfect commando roll onto the tube as the doors closed. She'd gone from the worst kind of person to a clumsy fool to my hero in a matter of seconds and she'll never know how much she means to me.'

* When it came to making this show I thought I would carefully select some themes that were carried between *Team Viking* and this and the final third show. The things I felt were important enough to me and the world include water, fire, animals, people being run over by emergency service vehicles, and McDonald's.

† This piece of music plays for longer than the others. It also has a G chord at the end which makes it feel complete.

‡ I describe whatever room we are currently in. This is my description of the Anatomy Lecture Theatre in Summerhall.

And Sarah and Emma walk in, they've been having the meeting with the registrar to confirm that they're humans and not, y'know, dogs or something. Music starts playing, Sarah and Emma stand at the front of the room,* just making it fucking weird. Just eyeballing everyone as the wedding march plays. It's great. They've decided they're both grooming each other because we talked about it and being a bride is shit, I mean being 'given away,' not being allowed to do a speech...dowries. I can only imagine that being a bride has become a typically emotionally febrile role culturally because of the immense amount of bullshit you have to put up with...almost like it's a metaphor for being a woman.

Giles there with his *atmosphere.* Sarah's nan singing along, there are no lyrics to the wedding march.

And the ceremony starts, we are welcomed and they do the legal bit, and it gets to the famous question. 'Does anyone present know of any just cause or impediment why these two people should not be married?'

Silence.

Suddenly the door slams open at the back, and standing there silhouetted in the entrance is

the Girl.

---

* 'Sarah and Emma had a long long argument over who was going to be the one who waited at the end of the aisle. In the end unfinished because they decided they'd both do it. Just play a piece of music at the beginning and that's it. Just both already be at the front. Together. In front of their friends and family. It sounded pretty good to me.'

Of course it is. I don't know if you've noticed, don't know if you've managed to read between the lines but she's always late, she always was, every time, didn't matter what the thing was, Sophie would always turn up later than she was supposed to. Always late, she –

Always.*

***

Her name is Sophie. Sorry.

I'm not going to tell you anything else about her because whatever you have imagined is better than I can describe to you in words.† Her name is Sophie. She's always late.

I always loved waiting for her.

And she creeps in at the back, sits down.‡ The registrar, entirely unflapped, continues and it's time for their vows and Emma goes first and she's memorised her vows, and

---

* The reaction of the reveal of her name is difficult to land. It depends so much on the set-ups and also really selling the Girl's arrival as if it's the main thing.

† For a while it was going to be that I described her at this point but differently every night: 'She's ____ tall, she has ____ eyes and ____ hair and she has a superpower; she listens. Really listens, all the time with everyone, it's nuts. Sometimes she misses train stops because she's listening to the announcements.'

‡ When I made the show for Vault Festival the Girl arrived at a nondescript moment in the ceremony. I felt like it was too melodramatic to use the obvious thing of it being at this point. Then just before Edinburgh I went to the wedding of my extraordinary friends Jonny and Wiggy. At exactly this point in the ceremony someone walked in, destroying the silence. It happened to also be the worst possible person to have interpolated. After that I had no choice.

they are perfect, beautiful, everyone in the room is warmed and smiling and with a single tear running down our face… wait, just me.* Now it is Sarah's turn and she takes a folded-up piece of paper out of her pocket, I'd asked if she wanted me to help her and she'd told me to go fuck myself. She starts to read: *Emma, I never thought that I'd get married, firstly because I thought that I wouldn't be allowed and then because I thought that nobody would want to and, and and…* and she's not stuck, she's crying, and it's really funny actually, actually no, no it's not funny. It's really bad. She's going red, oh God she was doing so well…it's all over. She can't speak at all, her mouth just opening and shutting like a landed fish. Emma's going red too, she's upset, she's angry and the registrar looks confused and Sarah's moving, she's leaving – No, she's edging towards me, she's grabbing my arm, she's pulling me up and she's passing me the paper…

'Do you want me to –?

Okay, I'll just carry on from…'

I take Sarah's hand.†

Emma, I never thought that I'd get married, firstly because I thought that I wouldn't be allowed and then because I thought that nobody would want to and even though I didn't want to do it like this (or with quite so many people here) now that I'm here I'm having quite

---

* This horrible line used to break up the narrative here: 'These fucking humans they're so great this is the best moment.'

† I have never performed this line. It occurred to me as I was re-editing the play for publication. I think it's good for the scene and also because it's echoing *Team Viking, and* because there's a bit near the end of *Revelations* where I'll be able to use it again.

a nice time (I wrote that bit down before because I knew it would be true) and that bit too, because I always have a nice time with you... and, and, and I've lost it, now I'm crying, I'm trying to stop but I can't see the words on the paper anymore and I've dropped it out... I'm gone I'm gone, I'm just a puddle on the floor and now Sarah is laughing and crying and so I'm crying and laughing and I've fucked it it's all fucked I can hear Emma saying 'stop it' and I can't, we can't and I can hear Giles grumble and get up and he's leaving, he's walking out – no –

He's walking to us. Straight towards us.

And he picks up the paper and he reads it beautifully:

'I'll just carry on as well.'

...I always have a nice time with you. And nice might seem a silly word, a little word, a word too small for a day like today but there's another meaning of it that people don't use very much anymore which is: proper, right, correct and that's what I mean. And I wish that Mum could have been here because she would have loved you...

'That's true Emma, she really would have.'

...and I promise I will always try and make things nice for you.

I was supposed to play a song that I'd written 'specially for the occasion while they signed the register but after that, no way. So instead we all sit in companionable quiet and smile, while Sarah and Emma sign a legally binding contract to their love which was what we all needed.

Giles was very funny actually: 'Does this mean we're all married now?'

'Yes Giles, yes it does.'

And we have a party, an incredible party, my only problem
with it is Sarah and Emma do the *Dirty Dancing* lift and neither
of them get hurt. Soph is here all the time, I don't talk to her
but I'm aware of where she is in the room all the time. All
the time… Sarah and Emma leave at midnight to go back to
Sarah's flat, their flat. They're not going on honeymoon for
a couple of weeks. It's late, and I'm standing at the bar and
Sophie's walking straight towards me and this time she really
is walking to me:

'Shall we go outside?'

'Yeah.'

We walk down the steps, and stand outside a window, the
lights and the shadows from the party flickering across our
faces. I smoke cigarettes, she might have had one, I can't
remember. We talk about how strange, how stupid, how great
everything is.

And now she's saying something but I can't hear her because
the million wriggling creatures in my stomach are screaming
at me to say what's on my mind –

'Soph, sorry Soph, sorry. I have to say, I just have to tell you
something…

I –

I miss you

I –

I'm really sorry

I –

I love you. I'm sorry, I love you."*

She said

'I know'

and she gave me a kiss, just here, so mainly beard but a bit of
lip. I'll take it. Then she got in a taxi and went home.

So.

So.

---

* 'I'm only half-listening to her some of the time, because I really want to
say something to her:
"Remember when we were driving to Center Parcs and we saw all those
lorries parked up with their doors open on the way? I found out why
that is. It's because the drivers have to have breaks, the engines cut out if
they go too long and so if their lorry is empty they leave the back doors
open to prove there's nothing inside so that no one tries to steal from
them and I think that's maybe how I was with you. That I was honest and
vulnerable and open…but I was asleep at the wheel. Sorry, sorry. That's
not what I want to say at all, that's not what I mean, what I want to say
is, I miss you. I love you. I'm sorry. I was so *stupid* of course I love you.
I love you."
I'm not going to tell you whether I said that or not. I can tell you that I really
wanted to and that when we finished talking she said 'I love you' and gave
me a kiss, just there, mainly beard. Then she got in a taxi and went home.'

I fucked Sarah's nan.*

Those hips don't lie. They can't, they're not old enough, they don't know what a lie is yet.†

No. We shared a Viennetta,‡ which if anything is sexier and more dangerous.

And then I called Sarah. I called my best friend on her wedding night. It went straight to answerphone.

I mime holding a phone.

'Hi this is Sarah (and Emma)' – in the background – 'we just got married so we won't be answering the phone for quite a while, unless this is you James. James, if this is you, the quilt's out on the sofa, we'll see you in the morning. You massive bellend.'

I mime throwing the phone up into the night sky where, after a few seconds, it explodes like a firework.

---

* This joke happened in an improv with my wonderful, brilliant, idiot friends Andrew Gruen and Amy Fleming (two of only three people I know who have missed Christmas because of a hangover). It was the first (and only) improv I've done drunk. Look. Okay. I take my work very seriously but I'd had a big night the night before and the only way I could face it was to have a drink. I'd got to this bit and the tone was *just so maudlin* and I felt self-conscious so made an inappropriate joke. It's the reason why I put 'a wordy cunt' in so readily – the quoting of an extreme swear word earlier makes this necessary crudity less severe.

† It occurs to me that I should put a bit in earlier about my nieces and them being three and one and not knowing what lies are in order for this stupid joke to land but if I carry on down that path I'll also have to mention Shakira.

‡ There was a bit: 'Sarah and Emma had realised that they could do whatever they wanted so we're all having Viennettas instead of a cake.'

Sometimes you need a sign, even if it's some flippant nothing, to help you realise that everything will be okay. Well I saw a tube mouse sitting on a Big Mac on my way.*

But none of this is true so it doesn't really matter does it.

I'd like to play the song I wrote for Sarah and Emma for you now.

I don't have the words for this
I don't know what to say
There's nothing I can do that could properly convey the way
I feel today

The world's too big for us and we can't cope cos we're too small
the only thing that'll get us through is our friends as we face it all.

But if I say that it sounds trite if I say I'm happy it's not quite
right, I haven't, haven't got the words.

Cos I'm just a boy singing for a girl...

And another girl, delighted by the way the worlds arranged for
us to celebrate change – cos

I don't like marriage much it's old-fashioned and it's out of touch
but that's been turned around by who you are,

From where I'm standing,

The sun's not just a star.

---

* Why are you still reading these? Why? I'm barely conscious. Go and live your life.

EASY PEELERS

Four shoes swept over the blue plastic floor as James and Sarah walked in silence down the quiet corridor. No longer needing signs, or coloured lines, following their feet, minds elsewhere. As they slowed to turn off the hallway Sarah put her hand on James' shoulder, he squeezed it back.

The antibac dispenser made a fart noise. James giggled at the same moment Sarah sighed, anticipating his juvenility. Their noises were so perfectly synchronised that Sarah couldn't help but join in with his laughter.

'I like your t-shirt.' The nurse greets them with a smile. 'Who are you here to see?'

'Pamela Attwood. Where's Orla?'

'She's moved to night shifts, you know where you're going then?'

'Thank you.'

They proceeded down the dingy little ward.

James opened a specific door and light fell out of it. Sarah walked in, he followed.

Sunlight smiled through the windows.

There was one completely remarkable thing about the room. It wasn't the two large windows taking up most of one wall. It wasn't the overbed table. It wasn't the food sat uneaten on the plastic tray on that table. It wasn't the door, ajar, and leading onto a wetroom with a toilet. It wasn't the hand basin or the sanitation station or the tall stern man sat up straight and quiet next to the bed, closing an old looking book on his lap. It wasn't the hand-knitted blanket over the hospital-issue sheets. It wasn't the tiny fragile woman, yellow skin paper thin, breath rattling, chest shuddering, half-sat up and sleeping underneath the blanket.

The room was covered in flowers.

In vases, in mugs, in glasses, one bunch of yellow roses in a cardboard bedpan; lined along the window sill, crowded on the bedside table, overflowing from the hand basin, and filling up every bit of floor that was not a thoroughfare. Variegated and verdant, as if a rainbow had found a solid form in room four of the Palliative Care Ward in St Anne's Hospital Northamptonshire, Great Britain, Europe, The Earth, The Solar System, The Universe, Existence.

James placed his bag at the foot of the bed between some chrysanthemums and an orchid.

'How long has she been out?' Sarah asked quietly, already arranging vegetable receptacles.

'An hour or so.' Giles, standing, stretching and tucking the book down the side of the chair's cushion. 'I'm going for a walk.' He opened his arms out awkwardly to his daughter. Sarah leant in and they shared a terrible, careful hug.

'You won't need your coat Dad, it's lovely out.'

'Right. Sure. Fine.' He took it off, folded it over the arm of the chair, nodded. 'James,' and wandered out of the room in shirtsleeves, looking for all the world like someone desperately looking for all the world.

'Is he okay?'

'He's okay.'

James played with some tulips. 'That was a weird hug mate.'

'Don't.' Sarah sneezed. 'Ugh.' She sneezed again.

'Bless you. How do you feel arranging the largest ever non-public display of cut flowers affects your hayfever on a scale of one to definitely?' James asked kindly, clearly genuinely interested in his friend's affliction, without a facetious bone in his body.

Sarah sneezed again, twice in quick succession.

'Bless you. Have you taken an antihistamine?'

'No.' Sneeze. 'Can I.' Sneeze. 'Have one.'

James fished out a little tin from his backpack, and fished out some piriteze from among the plasters and painkillers and handed them over.

Sarah took the sippy cup from the bedside table and swallowed two pills. Sneezed again and in doing so headbutted the beaker. 'Ow shit! James, it's gone in my eye James. Ow.'

James shook, helplessly laughing, dropping his bag which knocked over some lilies in a pint glass.

'You two are having fun.' The words punctured the laughter. The old lady's eyes had opened and somehow, behind the pain, a tiny, joyful constellation blazed.

Sarah threw herself into the chair 'Oh Nan I'm sorry, I'm a mess, I had some of your water and–' Sneeze. '–the flowers.' Sneeze. 'Did I wake you up?'

One frail hand found its way out from under the sheet and Sarah held it gently. 'It's nice to be awake. Where's your wife?' The words didn't come easily.

'Emma's working.' Sneeze. 'She gave us something for you.'

James looked up from sponging the floor with his jumper, took a parcel out of his backpack and held it out. Sarah's nan didn't move. 'I'll open it.'

He tore open the brown paper. Inside was a bag of easy peelers.

'Oh, lovely. May I have one?'

'Sure but I'm doing it under sufferance.'

Sarah explained between sneezes, 'James doesn't like them being called easy peelers.'

'Neither does Giles.'

'Well, that's probably different, I just really like satsumas and I think that this easy peeling thing will end up with us taking all of the diversity out of small oranges.' James spoke pompously as his thumb tore into the sunset skin in a familiar pattern. 'Anyway, there's already a perfectly good group name for them: mandarins.' The peel fell down on some poppies in one piece. 'Sorry. I just like satsumas.' He held the naked fruit towards her.

Sarah's nan gazed levelly at him. 'You are silly James.'

'Yes I am.' James smiled, arm outstretched, then realised in a flood of mortification she couldn't take the clementine off him, it had been days since she last ate anything at all. Helplessly he passed it to Sarah who frowned gently at him as she took it. Sneezed. 'Bless you.' And again. 'Bless you.' And again. 'Mate.' Sarah stood up still sneezing, she pressed the fruit back into his hand.

'I've got to get some –' Sneeze. '– air.' Sneeze. 'I'll see if I can find Dad.' Sneeze. She went out, opening and closing the door carefully and her sneezes echoed off the walls as they faded down the corridor.

Pam looked at James mildly. 'Can you rinse it? I don't want snot on it.'

'Sure.' He took it to the bathroom, no hand basin – of course, the sink sat in the main room and was therefore deputised as a flower pot. He switched on the shower managing to only half-soak his sleeve in the act of washing the orange. Shirt dripping he sat down, separated a segment. 'Will you be able to…?'

'I think so, you'll have to put it in my mouth and I'll try and suck on it.'

James felt…nothing actually. If there had been anyone else there he might have felt self-conscious, stupid even, but because he was alone with Sarah's nan there was no need for self-consciousness.

Pam sucked the segment through thin cracked lips, slowly, eyes closed. 'Lovely.'

'Would you like another?' The drip bag clicked and sighed as it released more drugs into her.

'No thank-you.' Eyelids fluttering, her sentence slightly broken, clearly hurting.

He took a tissue and wiped some errant juice from her chin.

'Do you want me to lie you back now?'

'No. Thank-you.'

'We watered your garden this morning. The roses are doing well, I think, well, they look like they're having a good time anyway. Your blackbird friend was looking for you. We tried to give her some toast like you did – like you do.' James corrected himself. 'But she wouldn't take it from us. She misses you.' He glanced over to see if she'd heard, but she was sleeping again, utterly relaxed, except for the stuttering rhythm of her chest and the rattle in her throat.

James fished out the book that Giles had secreted in the seat. Green canvas cover bleached by light, spine so faded that he couldn't read the print. He turned to the title page: *Peter and Wendy.* One of his favourite books. He flicked to the final chapter where the eternal child visits his friend who has grown ever so old. He read.

The sun shifted slowly in the sky, smiling on the pages of the story, smiling on Sarah and Giles talking together on a bench, smiling on a blackbird sitting lonely in a garden, smiling on kindness and cruelty and sadness and joy, smiling indiscriminately on every single thing that it could bloody smile on, smiling on the flowers that fed on its light.

'Giles reads that to me when he thinks I'm asleep.' Pam was awake and watching him, speaking slowly. 'I haven't told him I know, don't want to embarrass him.'

James, interrupted in the action of having his heart re-broken all over again by a tale he knew the end of, searched for something to say.

'I'm tired James. I don't want everything to stop, I don't want it to finish but I've had enough.' Every word being purchased from her pain at a prohibitive price.

There was nothing that he could say.

That didn't matter though, sometimes it's okay just to be there.

He held the part-eaten easy peeler in his left hand and her fragile little fingers in his right.

Eventually all of the flowers in the hospital room died. Eventually every living thing in that hospital room died. Eventually.

REVELATIONS

Set: Stage right a microphone, loop pedal and Casio keyboard sat on a bent-over music stand – not unlike a pulpit. Upstage centre an old amp with a folded piece of paper on it.

A pre-amble, talking about the venue/weather/my health/the attractiveness of the audience (always positive regardless of my feelings).

How's it going? I've got a favour to ask you before we begin. Right, I've got a niece and she's great and I love her and she loves me and I'm not very good at presents and I realised that I might be able to leverage the fact that I stand in front of people lots and get you to help me make a great present for her. So I've written the beginning of a song and I'm gonna ask every audience I perform to, to add bits to it, harmonies and it'll go on for as long as I keep doing this and then that'll be a really good present right? Is that okay?

Cool. So it goes like this:

I teach them the tune one line at a time.

'The world is so big and we are so small'

    Great

'And sometimes it is hard to make sense of it all'

    Lovely

'But I love you and I'll be here'

    Excellent

'And some day Lydia we'll go for a beer'

Now let's practise that all together.

Amazing that's brilliant, now we'll go for a take which those of you in 'the business' will know there is traditionally only one of.

I pick up a recording device and speak into it.

Hello Lydia, it's Uncle Jim here, me and some of my future friends are going to sing you a song, one, two, three:

The world is so big and we are so small,
And sometimes it's hard to make sense of it all,
But I love you and I'll be here,
and someday Lydia we'll go for a beer.

A beer is like a juice but better.

I stop the recording.

Thank you very much.

Right.

Now, I'll go and do the lights and when I come back I'll be a performer and all the rest of this will be artifice.

Hello. My name is James. I'm going to tell you a story.

I call upon God the Father, God the Son and God the Holy Spirit to aid me in this account.

***

Music One.

No one knows why we love music. Our bodies respond to music by releasing dopamine which is a reaction usually reserved for things we need like sex, or food, or Facebook.

I love singing, on my own or with other people. I feel like the collective act of communion fulfils something fundamental.

And everyone can sing, maybe not in tune, but when you sing with other people the stronger voices carry the weak and together you are reaching for something further, something higher, something beyond ourselves.

***

Pure white clots of cotton wool drifted down and settled silently on the warm grey city; making London look less like a messy metropolis teeming with inequality and ideas, but rather, a half-finished sketch of somewhere beautiful by some slow-working celestial artist.

When I woke up I just knew. A different quality of the light around my curtains and the absolute quiet of outside.

It never snows in London, well, clearly it does, but not enough because snow is the best. I don't find anything more ratifying of the life choices I've made to avoid adult responsibility than it snowing because I can instantly guarantee that Uncle Jim is having a snow day. Its levelling effects are amazing, some of the simplest, happiest most fun moments of my life have been in snow in London. Homeric Snowball fights with strangers, Snow people made with friends, sledging down Parliament Hill at terrifying speeds next to a very old man gently descending on an old bit of carpet.

So I immediately texted Emma and Sarah. Emma replied that being a 'Human Rights Lawyer means not having snow days – open brackets – you fucking idiot – close brackets – pub later.'

Sarah didn't respond, I imagine she was too busy doing… her job (she's my best friend, I've known her for my entire life and I feel like it's her business, I respect her privacy. I have a don't ask, don't ask policy because I think it's boring). So I sent out messages to all my self-unemployed friends. Which was a *staggering* insight into the snares of a capitalist existence because they all had something to do. Like someone was having an infected neck piercing removed, someone else had a legitimate medical complaint being seen to (they've asked me not to share it with you anymore but it was Rob and gonorrhoea), most gallingly one couple were viewing houses.

So I had to lone wolf it and let me tell you experience of playing in the snow as an adult man is very different when you're not with a friendly looking group of friends. You appear, in fact, to be a Lone Wolf. Cos I'd be like:

Mime throwing snowball at someone and them not liking it and running away.

And doing a snow angel on your own for yourself is about the saddest thing it's possible to do… I made a big snow dick though – it wasn't supposed to be that – I didn't go, 'Heeey it's phallus time.' I just started making something and y'know, the snow chooses, I am merely the channel of its intention.

So I was on my way home after frankly a very disappointing snow day and something made up for it entirely because as I went past the primary school at the end of my road the foxes who live underneath the playground were performing a mummers play of my life. There was this tiny perfect fox cub just dancing, just *dancing* overjoyed by the newness of the snow, and getting really close to me – cos the thing is foxes learn to be afraid of human beings and this one was just too, too young to care about the shabby man entranced by their innocence. Right there just dancing. Then I spotted two older foxes under shelter on the other side of the playground watching us – probably planning a mortgage.

I went home, got warm (had a bath) and went out about nineish to meet Sarah and Emma at the pub. We always have to meet later because Emma's a human rights lawyer and I don't want to explode anyone's mind with too much truth but have you noticed that the better your job is for the world the worse it is for you.

Mime someone's head exploding.

Yeah. I see you: Nurses, Doctors, Actors.

Someone had to call it, if not me, when? If not now, who?

I got to our local (we've got a local, very grown up) and they were there and they were being *weird*. They were waiting for me at the bar (which they never do) to buy me a drink (which was even stranger). Then we got our favourite table by the fire and they sat opposite me like they were about to conduct an audition (job interview).

I was immediately worried, I didn't know how I'd upset them but I felt like I had. You'd think aged thirty-one (as I was at the time) I'd have known that I'm okay with people, especially my closest friends, but all that my experience has taught me is the vast amount of variables that exist in every human being so you can never really know what someone's actually thinking. So I was quite panicked, I was like:

'I'm really sorry, was it the text where I compared you to Herod cos I was just joking cos you didn't come and pl–'

'No, actually James–' Emma she's older than me and Sarah and she bullies me, in a friend way. She comments on my quiddities from atop her high horse. She is married to Sarah, who's been my best friend forever, she's an idiot. Two PhDs but that's easy right? Must be if she's got them.

'No, actually James. The reason we want to talk to you is we've been discussing something for a while and we wanted to tell you.

We've decided we're going to start a family.'

'You're going to what?'

'We're going to have a baby.'

'A what?

'A baby.'

…

…

'What about me? I thought I was your baby, who's going to look after me?'

'The thing is James' (Sarah) 'we thought what with you being thirty-one you'd be able to look after yourself.'

'Well that was pretty presumptuous of you wasn't it I'm barely allowed matche–'

'That's not all James, and I need you to know this goes against every rational fibre of my being but we really love you. And we're wondering if you, if you would want to, if you would like to be the sperm donor.'

Childish snort of laughter

'Oh you're not joking. Oh. Oh? You're not going to adopt, I assumed you'd be adopti – ah but I see how that is a stupid thing to say.'

'No, it's not actually, we've talked about that a lot and we might in the future, we want more than one child but thing is, Emma really wants to carry a baby. So do I, actually –'

'But I'm older, so my eggs get first crack.'

'You don't have to answer straight away.'

***

Music Two.

Sarah moved in next door to me when we were five years old and instantly we became inseparable, together with our friend Tom we terrorised our parents, our schools and especially our church. A warm and welcoming community that cared for us and protected us from the extremities of modern childhood. I loved Sarah from the moment that we met.

Tom was a creature of pure excitement, a hurricane of adventure. Often I felt like a sapling bent low beneath the force of his storm but when Sarah arrived, there was another sapling: more deeply rooted than I was and together we were able to stand the force of Tom's rambunctious wind. I loved Sarah for that with the fierce joy of the young.

Every night before I went to sleep Mum or Dad (who at that point in my life went by the names of Mummy and Daddy) would pray with me, a meditative way to finish the day, relinquishing my worries and sending them up to God to deal with overnight. Obviously my requests varied from day to day but the first four words never wavered 'Dear Lord Jesus, Please...'

After I met her my first request sent up was set in stone: 'Dear Lord Jesus, please look after Sarah.'

***

I said yes because they promised me I'd have no responsibility after the initial input, because the law in fact enshrines that, they're married so legally I would have no commitment, because I knew they would be incredible parents because I love them and because I wanted to.

So I had to make a deposit in the Bank of Semen. You've heard of it? Obviously the interest rates are slightly skewed post-Brexit but I still think it's safer than cryptocurrency and remember it's all legal tender, so don't let any taxi drivers talk you out of using it...

Now I'm not going to go on about it too much as I don't want to make any of the gentlemen in the audience feel insecure but buckle up because my sperm is *absolutely* average. Nothing clever down there, I'm not gonna lie I was sort of hoping that it would be shit. You know, the way that you can be extra cool by undermining what's normally good like:

'My guys swim in circles actually,' rather than, 'Hey I'm super fertile.'

You know like friends who say their favourite Shakespeare play is *Cymbeline*. Or self-identifying as a Hufflepuff.

So my spunk's motility is neither feast nor famine. Neither wheat nor chaff. Just a light meal. Workable. Ooh I had such a good time when I handed little pot of cum over to the nurse Michael, I was grinning my head off, like: 'Isn't this amazing!' He found my enjoyment very disconcerting. I was just thinking: 'This is literally your job!'

That was my work discharged... Back to the normal lifelong friendship.

The method they were using was IUI in case you are a layman. Which is exactly how it doesn't work, crucially no men are laid at all.

IUI not IVF. Inter Uterine Insemination not In Vitro Fertilisation. So it's Insemination rather than Fertilisation an it happens Uterus rather than a vitro and we all know what a Vitro is. A type of car. The Ford Vitro...

Cars are strange aren't they. I had my first ever panic attack because of cars. I mean my girlfriend had left me, my Dad had died and my best friend had died but I'm preetty sure it was the cars that set me off. I was waiting at a train station for Sarah to pick me up and there was this multi-story thing there, and it was just too much. They're incredibly expensive, they're completely destroying the planet, after ten years or something you just throw them away and they can kill people. I mean obviously cars don't kill people, people kill people. (Well done James, you tell it right, get on that bandwagon.) But it's astonishing the mental acrobatics we'll perform to allow ourselves the label of normal. The idea that piloting a one ton lump of metal around is *normal?* It's a phenomenal leap of faith that is carried out on a daily basis by billions of people, many of whom I'm sure wouldn't credit themselves with any unusual level of imagination.

IUI not IVF. IUI is very similar to the classic heterosexual technique but you don't use a willy because they are notoriously unreliable.

We still met up in the pub all the time although neither of them were drinking (Sarah staunchly in support was doing everything that Emma was, the diet, not drinking, tracking her cycle).

The first attempt went by. Nothing happened.

Then the second, still…

And the third attempt was coming up which was a big deal because Emma had decided that was going to be it. Three strikes and you're out, because she was now thirty-seven – not the album, but old enough to remember the album and the bangers therein contained – and I thought that was very sensible because it's an impossibly hard decision to make but it has to be made. How long can you just stay in stasis, literally waiting for life to happen.

So there was a lot of pressure on it.

By the way, I've asked Emma at every stage if it is okay for me to tell this story and share this stuff and she's always said yes.

Emma had in her teenage years, two late term abortions. Every abortion you have makes your chance of conceiving considerably smaller. So unfair...the whole thing is. There are these people; kind, caring willing people who find it impossible to make a baby while people who don't want to have the 'gift of life' thrust on them to live with or abort, fucking teenagers who'd rather get Chlamydia than a baby and they end up having both.

About a week or so after the third attempt I got a text from Sarah saying 'let's meet early in the pub today'. Absolutely.

When I turned up at the pub they were at our table they were drinking, they were laughing – my heart exploded:

'Guys! Congratulations!'

They turned to me, faces ashen. I'd called it so badly wrong.

It hadn't worked.

They were laughing because sometimes you just laugh.

And I sat down and we all had a good cry together. Well they had a good cry. I didn't cry, I never cry.

I'm very brave.

And one of the minor miracles about pubs worked its magic. We have these public houses, where people afford each other privacy. People left us to our peculiar grief but they were still there. We were in a place where community invisibly cradles the personal.

The thing Sarah kept on repeating was the thing the doctor had said to them: 'Everything works better when you're younger.'

Everything works better when you're younger.

So we got drunk. We got really drunk. I'm want to make that totally clear and then draw a line underneath it because being drunk isn't an excuse for anything. It can be a reason, we had a lot of reasons, pints and pints of reasons.

And it got to the point of no return (when you're guaranteed a hangover so you might as well crack on).

'Guys, why don't we go back to my house and get Sarah pregnant tonight, I've got Pernod, let's make a baby.'

And they went for it!?

We got back to my place: I poured us all a pastis, enchanté. I changed my sheets – monsieur – and went to the salle de bains to get ready.

I took all my clothes off. Now it has been a while since I've felt like taking gland in hand in a bathroom – a while since I *just couldn't wait*. I couldn't sit on the edge of the bath because it was sharp on my bum and the floor was this very cold hard Mexican ceramic tile, there was nothing happening, after a few minutes' fruitless failure I went to tell them –

Emma screamed and Sarah was cowering against the wall. 'James! Put some clothes on, you're naked, you're naked!'

'Oh! Oops. Sorry. That's quite funny.'

'It is not funny.'

'Look, I'm really sorry and I don't want make it weird, but just nothing's happening.'

'James, are you using porn?'

'No! I want it to be special.'

'James take my phone, put on some porn and go and do what have to do.'

'Wank in the bathroom.'

'Yes.'

'Oh and James.' Sarah called me back 'Put some clothes on before you come back in because, and I want to be very clear about this, *I'd rather die than ever see you naked again.*'

So I did what I had to do. Into a pint pot that I'd liberated from our local. I took it through and left them too it. Apparently though Emma used a bar spoon, which, obviously, very practical and thematically on point.

I wanna be very clear that that was the last time I've ever handed anyone a receptacle of my semen.

Except for one lucky audience member tonight.

Thank-you for contributing on Kickstarter.

***

Music Three.

Tom, Sarah and I grew up in a church family, it really was a kind of family as everyone took care to be there for one another. The fact that there are things you can mock in religion shouldn't undermine the genuine love and care that exists there. It's very easy to patronise belief, but don't throw the baby out with the bathwater, I mean it is funny, of course there are things that are funny, that's the nature of human existence; we are ridiculous creatures often when we are being most serious and that applies to religion or sex or alcohol or gardening or death.

In our church, there was a belief that you could pray for and receive the gift of speaking in tongues. I'll lay it out for you: Jesus is back in heaven and God sends the Holy Spirit to the disciples to give them gifts so that they could spread the gospel. The primary gift was the ability to speak all languages – the gift of speaking in tongues. This event was called Pentecost.

Now the structure of a church service is very close to that to the structure of a one-person show (if I've made it). Welcome, song, prayer, song, reading, song, sermon, song, prayer.

One evening service when we were thirteen years old took Pentecost as its theme. So the prayer at the end was for the gift of speaking in tongues.

If you wanted to be prayed for you went and stood at the front and the prayer ministry team would gather around, that night it went like this:

I mime the ministry team laying on hands and the person being prayed for.

'Hamanahanshamanana'

'Loiskapoiskaroskamashaposj'

'Wasofadwasofdijababafewijowfe'

Somewhere on the spectrum of baby talk/Ringwraiths/Louis Armstrong.

After a couple of minutes of this Tom got up and walked to the front for prayer. (I should be clear, aged thirteen Tom had already decided his biblical path was to be that of the serpent. With a ruthless logic I'm still in awe of to this day he was like 'I don't wanna practise Christianity, I wanna practise sex.' But he still came to church with us because there's nothing else to do on a Sunday night when you're thirteen, besides, he badly wanted to uproot Sarah and I.)

Tom got up and walked to the front. The Vicar looked slightly concerned, but Tom assumed the position, eyes closed hands upturned. The ministry team gathered around.

I take the character of Tom.

'Ski-bob

…

Ski bag bob bidabob
Ski ba dibby dib yo da dub dub
Yo da dub dub

Ski-bi dibby dib yo da dub dub
Yo da dub dub'

He was the scatman. The whole church got up and started dancing… Well no. Tom and Sarah and I were in a lot of trouble.

***

So Sarah's pregnant. You got that right? You know how stories work.

Now, I'm here to tell you legends that pregnancy is amazing. Seriously. It's someone, growing someone inside them. Genuinely I had completely underestimated it before. I think largely because of the language associated with it being devalued words like 'miracle' and phrases like 'gift of life' being used without any awe or wonder. Used pejoratively, politicised, as sticks to wound people, without the worth and wonder those words should carry.

I wanted to be as useful as possible so I read lots of books about pregnancy, I made sure I was available, I took up yoga… The books were fascinating, I learned all sorts of stuff – like waters breaking, that's not a real thing, well, it is a real thing but it's not what starts most labours, it's just a visual cue that Hollywood has cottoned on to.

The only thing that was properly useful though was taking Sarah McDonald's, she got these mad craving for McDonald's, I said

'Interestingly cravings aren't a real thing –'

'Shut up James, get me the burger.'

Now while pregnancy is incredible, it lasts *foreeeever*. Literally (it's still in there), no. So long. The watched pot, the drying paint. Boring.

So I'll skip forward to the twelve week scan. Parents were told, Emma's parents delighted, Sarah's dad Giles confused:

'I just don't understand why you had to use his sperm when you could have had an astronaut's.'

'The thing is Dad we just want to have a terrifically hairy baby.'

And then again, up to the twenty week scan, back to waiting, like watching a tree grow. I mean, there was a little bump, more McDonald's (there was one halfway between our flats so I'd stop off and pick up dinner on my way over to theirs, next door to the Rose and Crown, we had replaced locals). I was staying over, being there, hanging out.

The twenty week scan was a big day, a huge day. I woke up on their sofa that morning and it had snowed, oh yeah, two years in a row. Someone up there must love me (even if it's a hole in the ozone layer). It was amazing and terrifying and awful because I had responsibilities. I had to wait in their flat to take delivery of a crib. Promised delivery between 8 a.m. and 12 in the afternoon whichever one it is I never know and it was late, delayed and I just spent the whole day pacing around the flat like a caged tiger. Like a caged bear. Like a caged man-child. Occasionally going to the window and seeing people just scorning the snow as they walked past, it took all of my resolve not to shout at them:

'ROLL AROUND! IT WON'T BE THERE IN THE MORNING! YOU ARE WASTING THE SNOW! YOU ARE WASTING YOUR LIFE!'

Eventually the flat pack arrived but it was dark so I left it in the corner and stomped home, feeling really annoyed actually...

I got home and realised it was six-thirty which means they'd have had the scan by now.

I've noticed that when you're in a new context that has an existing social silhouette, regardless of how resilient you think you are, the simplest step is to subscribe to the structure that's already there. So despite the three of us considering ourselves as an alternative brook rather than any part of the main stream we were really excited about finding out the biological sex of the baby. It's really not something any of us generally consider important but the edifice exists and we walked into it. Excited.

I waited for them to call me, text me, tell me what the news was. Nothing. So about eight I went fishing. I texted Sarah.

'McDonald's?'

'Absolutely. The usual.'

I put my coat on and left and something magical happened.

One of the foxes from the primary school started following me. I could only imagine my accidentally dropping drunken fast food purchases on my way home had finally paid off. I just had a sense, because they were quite small, that they must be my buddy from last year's snow day. I knew I couldn't look at them directly because they'd get spooked but they was definitely following me, breath pooling in the air. I got to

McDonald's, ordered the usual (two Big Macs, twenty chicken nuggets), Sarah's stuff.

I came out and they were still there, watching, waiting over the road. Let's dance. So I walked past the Rose and Crown, down the street towards Emma's and Sarah's just to see if... and they did. Their shadow surreptitiously slipping between parked cars opposite. I decided to make a move, dropping a handful of chicken nuggets steaming on the snowy pavement and moving on until I paused on the corner. Back turned. Affecting un-interest.

Out of the furthest corner of my eye I see their dark shape, the other side of the road, they poke their head out, sniff the air then, finally, smoothly stepping from the snowy pavement onto the slush of the street. Holding my breath as they tiptoe across cautiously, softly, gently.

Then, suddenly, from nowhere, bright blue light in the other corner of my eye, streaming round the corner super-fast. I wheel around. 'Mate watch out watch out.' The fox freezes. In terror, in confusion and the police car flashed between us and the road is empty. The fox had gone. They'd gone.

No. No, no, no, no. A small dark shape on the other pavement further down. Not moving. I ran across the road, which was stupid because I didn't look and you must always look you never know and there it was on the pavement. Somewhere in between the car flashing between us it had stopped being a they and become an it. Perfect. Beautiful. The only sign of something wrong were its sightless eyes and blood bright red trickling from its mouth into the snow around its head.

And I decided it couldn't be my buddy, my snow day friend. It couldn't be it had to be different, there's no – and I wanted to commemorate it somehow – you'd think with a lifetime of Christianity I would know…but there isn't any liturgy for roadkill. And I got a text from Sarah saying:

'I've got news for you if you've got McDonald's for me.'

So I left it. Left it on the street. Walked away. Picked up the McDonald's, dusted the snow off it and carried a weird atmosphere as well as enormous amount of fast food to their house.

I got there, took a deep breath and let myself in. There they are on the sofa ready, waiting for me excitedly. They told me: it's a boy.

'I've got some ideas, hear me out, I was thinking: James – coz obviously both of you're gonna change your names, you'll be Mummy or Mum, obviously Emma you'll be Mammah. So I thought I could maybe be Uncle Jim so you can call him James and it won't be confusing.'

Emma said, 'No actually we've already decided what we're going to call him. We're gonna call him Tom.'

Which stopped me in my tracks because there's a reason why our childhood friend Tom isn't around anymore. He died aged twenty-five. Some of you will know that because I've told the story before. It had been Emma's suggestion and it was amazing because Sarah and I still bear those scars, and like any scars they still hurt sometimes. The name seemed like a good, healing thing. And it was actually after that day that things got brilliant. Because like any two trees planted close together Sarah and I have grown up and around and through and in and out of each other, sharing each other's sunlight and drinking the same rain but you have to give a friendship time as well and it was after this we started to have that time. Emma picked up a big court case, you might have read about it in the papers: securing the rights of refugee children to be patriated to this country, to join their families. She tried to get all the prep done as much as possible so she could be around for Ma/Paternity Pa/Maternity – we didn't ever settle on the right one. So she was leaving the house before six she was getting home after midnight and Sarah was tired so I'd go round in the evening, hang out with her and then I'd wait up for Emma and fill her in on the evening.

But then Sarah got to maternity leave and it was even better, we had acres to grow into, whole days to hang out. We watched all the old films: *Vikings*, *When Harry Met Sally*, the Disney *Robin Hood* (which I found very traumatic though I didn't explain why). Then we watched ones to get us ready for the baby: *Junior* (at which point I realised that I'd very much been working on a sympathetic pregnancy my entire life), *Three Men and a Baby*, *Three Men and a Little Lady*, *Alien*. All the stuff that we needed and it was getting very close to B-day (not bathroom refurbishment, the birth-day. Time. They had a bag of stuff sitting ready to take to hospital). And I woke up to an empty flat – Sarah had gone to visit her dad, she went to visit Giles because they didn't want him visiting too soon after the baby arrived. Emma had arranged to get the evening off when Sarah got back. So when I awoke I tidied the whole flat so it'd be really nice for them when they got back. Their first evening off together for months. As I finished and was about to leave I saw the crib still flat-packed against the wall in the living room... Uncle Jim.

Now I'm gonna pause the show for a minute and make a genuine offer. If anyone doesn't like doing flat pack furniture my twitter handle is @jdsrowland, yeah. I'll pay for my own transport, two requests (rules): one, I make my own tea. Two, you have to let me alone because I don't like any of that.

I mime someone chatting in my ear.

But honestly do hit me up.

So I made it and it was brilliant I had nailed it and I left and went to the gig I had that evening and I didn't switch my phone back on until I was on the train on the way home. And my screen filled up: Message, message, message, missed call, missed call, missed call, Sarah Sarah, Sarah. Oh no.

'Oh mate please tell me you're not at your dad's house, please tell me you made it back to London. Which Hospital are – actually you're probably not in hospital – how dilated are you? Sarah?

Sarah?'

...

And then a tiny voice at the other end:

'Emma's gone.'

They'd come home they'd seen –

They'd seen the crib.

The crib had been the final straw for Emma, it all came gushing out.

She felt excluded completely. She felt cut off. She felt like she was nothing to do with her baby. This resentment built in her and she had no way of expressing – She'd been busy, she'd been busy trying to look after some other children. Trying to be ready for –

She said 'It doesn't even feel like my baby, it feels like your baby with James.'

Sarah had defended me and Emma had gone. Her phone was off. I got back to their flat and found Sarah shattered. In pieces on the floor and exhausted because you can only cry so much. I got her to bed, she shook herself to sleep and then I sat up on the sofa waiting for Emma. Waiting for Emma to come home so I could fix it.

I must have fallen asleep.

***

Music Four.

Between the ages of fourteen and sixteen, Sarah and I went to the Christian Rock Festival: Soul Survivor. Has anyone else been?

If someone in the audience has:

Yeah! That's what I'm taking about! We walk among you.

If the rest of you think that that sounds uncool you are halfway there: it is phenomenally uncool.

But actually, that's not the problem with it because fuck coolness. Coolness doesn't care, coolness isn't kind, cool is cool. Give me warmth.

Tom had come once – our first time when we were fourteen, and had vowed never to return but Sarah and I returned the two subsequent years, when we were sixteen it felt like it had come at the right time. Sarah had found out her mum was ill, breast cancer, the prognosis was really good but it was still huge, horrible news. I was really proud of how brave she was being but worried nonetheless, I thought maybe the week would help.

We arrived, put up our tent and went to sleep in our separate compartments. I woke up the next morning with the worst knowledge I've ever woken up with in my life.

Music stops.

I woke up knowing that I was in love with Sarah. This flame inside me, fiercer than anything I'd ever felt before. A fire that threatened to burn down our entire forest.

So I got up, threw some clothes on and I left, I spent the whole day away from anywhere that Sarah might go: basket weaving, drum circles – both of which were great, I went to the big evening service and stood way away from where we usually were. She still saw the though, she managed to find me in the crowd so I had to run, I lost her and I lost myself. I spent the whole night away from our campsite away from our tent. I met some kind strangers (Christians can stay up late too you know) and it was one of those halcyon heatwave summers as all of them are in my memory but this one actually was, so I could sleep outside.

Then the next day again, time away from anywhere Sarah might go, I went to the talk about masturbation being sinful or wives submitting to their husbands or homosexuality being evil…yeah it's not the un-coolness that's not cool. I went to the evening service that night and the theme of it was Lazarus so the prayer at the end was for healing. I had never felt the need for healing more than I did on that night, so I stepped forward. I went and stood at the front and some kind strangers got up.

I motion to some people on the front row – give them whatever encouragement they need to get involved.

They laid their hands on me. One of them was praying in tongues.

They pray in tongues.

A bit louder than that actually.

They pray louder.

For ages.

They continue.

And actually, I felt really moved because I understood properly for the first time what speaking in tongues is really about. It's about the places where there are no words the spaces between them and of course it's silly but these people didn't know me, they didn't know what I was praying for, they didn't know what I wanted to be healed of but they made a decision to try and intercede on my behalf. I found it really moving.

And I knew the response I should be having. When the Holy Spirit works you get knocked down by the power of the lord… but nothing was happening, so after a few minutes fruitless failure I decided that I'd fake it because I wanted to reward them, reward their selfless gesture. So I started to rock backwards and forwards (because I wasn't entirely confident they'd catch me).

And they got ready to catch me.

And they lowered me back all the way, gently to the floor.

One of them found my jumper and put it carefully under my head. Squeezed my shoulder gently and left me alone.

I say the last line so they know to leave. Usually the audience applauds them but I never encourage it.

***

I woke up to the sound of the door slamming – where. Oh shit, no, Sarah. But as I ran to the front door I saw she was still in her bed, fists tightly curled, still asleep. It must have been Emma oh god. I ran to the door but I was too late. I got to the window in time to see her disappearing around the corner. Oh god. She'd come back. She'd seen me and she'd gone again.

I couldn't sleep it was five in the morning so I waited for Sarah to wake up and she started calling everybody. Called Emma's parents, they'd not heard. She'd called in sick to work so I left to look for her. I went everywhere she might go, all the cafes in the area, the library, McDonald's. I walked round the park for hours and I couldn't see her, couldn't find her, eventually I thought maybe the pub? That's where I'd go. So I went to the pub and she was there. Sitting at our table waiting for me.

Of course I laid it all out, apologised, I was –

She stopped me mid-sentence. Explained of course there was nothing she could do, she said:

'What do you want me to say James? It's alright? It's not alright. Nothing's going to change what's happened. You want me to say I forgive you? I don't. I will forgive you. I love you but it's hurting too much now. That's not the point.'

That wasn't the point. I was not the point.

Now sometimes a problem can be the size of a country, sometimes it can be the size of a car (three thousand six hundred people a day and half of the foxes in this country find cars a terminal problem). Sometimes they can be the size of one human brain, one human heart.

Emma couldn't bear it. Which is a horrible pun. There was no way she could have conceived of the way she felt but when Sarah got pregnant, this thing started growing inside Emma. Jealousy. Anger? Disappointment, mortification at her own body and most of all just rage, fury at herself for feeling that way.

I was sitting on the other side of the table from her as she just dredged bucket after bucket of woe from this bottomless well and poured them out over the table.

Suddenly her face changed – I knew why as soon as her eyes flicked up behind me – she'd seen a familiar silhouette out of the corner of her eye. Sarah was there, huge in the doorway.

'Mate, I'm so sorry, I just got here, I found her. I was going to call you any second –'

'James shut up, it's not about you. Emma, where have you been?'

'I stayed at James' house this morning –'

'Oh yeah, you've got keys –'

'– shut up James! Emma, please tell me what's going on?'

'I can't Sarah, I can't.'

'Emma, you have to tell me what's going on because I love you and I'm carrying our baby.'

And as she said 'our' something about it, I don't know what it was. It hit Emma. It hit her. I could see it light up her face from the inside out. She lit up and then started sobbing. Then she realised she was crying in a pub and she *does not like public stuff.* So she started laughing at herself. Then Sarah started laughing as well and when you're heavily pregnant your pelvic floor has absolutely gone to shit so she pissed herself.

I was like, 'Don't worry about it mate because when you're heavily pregnant your pelvic floor is –'

And she was like, 'Shut up James.'

Emma was like, 'Was that your waters breaking?'

Sarah was like, 'Uh-huh, that was my waters breaking.'

I was like, 'Your waters have broken!'

The whole pub went:

The audience cheer (hopefully).

Probably out of relief that we weren't shouting at each other anymore.

I was like, 'Oh the baby's coming, the baby's coming, okay okay. The baby's coming. Do you still want me around?' (I was going to be the extra birth partner.)

'Of course go and get the bag.'

'Go and get the bag! Of course, I'm going, I'm going!'

I run in one direction off stage, then back across the other way shouting.

'It's not at my house, it's definitely not at my house.' Then I had to sort of fast walk a lot of the way cos I am NOT VERY HEALTHY, so it was some time before I got back to the pub and stuff had really accelerated. Now I'm going to be using some quite graphic language over the next few minutes, if anybody doesn't like it just hold the hand of the person responsible for you being here and remember your breathing exercises.

The contractions were coming think and fast and Sarah was already like five centimetres dilated. Scout's Honour.

I hold up the Scouts three fingers.

So we had to get her to the hospital. I called an Uber. It arrived I got in the front seat they got in the back, she said: 'Are they going to be okay?'

I replied 'Don't worry about that, what's it like being a female Uber driver?' Just really fascinated by the female experience while my friend was mid-labour on the back seat.

We got to the hospital, handed over the notes, met our midwife. She was called Paula. I fancied her…which I'm not proud of but full disclosure. I really fancied her. We got our room and childbirth is similar to pregnancy in that this feels like it lasted for seconds in my memory but actually it was hours. Things were ticking along…

'I'm gonna get myself a cup of tea. Emma, Sarah, do you want – no, that's fine. Paula do you want anything? Coffee? Maybe you'll want one.'

I went and got the hot drinks, came back in.

'I got you a coffee. I'll just put it here.' Now Sarah was finding it quite a lot easier if she had her contractions standing up.

Paula must have decided she wanted the coffee at some point because Emma had gone to the loo so Sarah had grabbed her during a contraction and the coffee was spilling, it was spilling on the floor. Then I saw the coffee still sitting on the side and realised that wasn't coffee on the floor.

That was blood.

Falling out of Sarah.

Splashing on the floor.

Paula had seen it as well because she was already helping Sarah back to the bed and she must have hit a button or pulled a chord because by the time that Emma got back there were eight other nurses there and a woman (who if you cut her in half would have the word 'matron' written through her) issuing short, reassuring orders to everybody.

Emma asked what was going on.

'I don't know, I don't know she's bleeding a lot.'

You could see, between Sarah's legs on the sanitary surface of the table expanding on the cotton pads like blood in the snow. The matron came to us:

'Sarah's bleeding a lot more than I'm happy with.'

A man came in a few minutes later. He examined Sarah, had a brief word with the matron then he came over to Emma and I:

'So Sarah is bleeding a lot more than is normal, a lot more than is safe in fact. I have to tell you that there is a chance that we will lose the baby. We may also lose Sarah.'

I walk over to the microphone and repeat those words into the loop pedal.

'There is a chance that we will lose the baby. We may also lose Sarah.'

It repeats as I walk back centrestage and lie down in the same position as I was when the interceding audience members left me, I fade the music out and lie there.

Now. I didn't know the right amount of time to stay lying on the floor when you've been struck down by the power of the

Lord. So I just hung out until I felt like nobody was paying me any attention. I sat up (slowly so I didn't get dizzy) and sitting right in front of me was Sarah.

'I'm not surprised you needed a nap James, you can't have got much sleep last night.'

'Yeah... Look mate, I really need to tell you something.'

'I need to tell you something too James.'

She helped me up and we walked out of the tent and up the hill opposite, threading our way between other pairs and small groups of young Christians having life-changing conversations.

We stood at the top of the hill.

'You go first.'

'No, you go first James.'

'I said first –'

'Alright... Look, I think you know what I'm gonna... You're going to make me say it? Alright. James... I'm gay.'

'– I know.'

I said I know before a single thought had run through my head because I knew. I knew, I'd always known. We always, I mean of course. Of course. It had never been said before. It had never – this huge unspoken truth sat on her shoulders like an unbearable weight. Between us. The second that she said it was an incredible relief and the romantic feelings that I thought I'd felt for her over the previous thirty-six hours vanished like a raindrop in the ocean.

'I know.'

'I thought so, that's why you've been avoiding me, you, you worked it out.'

'No! Oh mate no of course not, that's not what it is at all.'

'Well what is it then?'

…

I don't know why but somehow in her saying something that had been so obvious and so unspoken another thing we knew, I knew, was new, had found crystal clarity.

'Oh. I don't believe any of this. None of it. I don't think I ever have.'

'That's quite good actually James because I'm definitely going to hell now, it doesn't matter how much you pray for me.'

'Well, I'd never pray for you anyway.'

'Every night. Tom told me.'

'Yeah. Well, I'm never gonna pray for you ever again.'

I go back and turn the loop pedal back up.

'There is a chance that we will lose the baby. We may also lose Sarah.'

Loop turns off.

Standing there in the antiseptic room, time treacled. I watched Emma float over to Sarah, stroke her head, and out of nowhere Sarah's face turned and her eyes locked on mine. She looked at me. Pleading, desperate, really afraid and I had nothing.

I needed to pray, I had to, I couldn't do anything else...but I couldn't pray and somewhere from the flickbook of memory racing through the back of my mind one image stuck. Where this had started, where it had begun, but I remembered Sarah looking up at me and saying:

'James, I'd rather die than ever see you naked again.'

And I had my t-shirt and shoes off before any of the nurses had noticed and then they looks aghast at me for about half a second before going back to the important stuff they were doing and then my trousers were off and I was still focusing right on Sarah. Then I had my pants off and there I was naked, staring at my friend in her hospital room and I swear, I swear I saw the shadow of a smile on her face before she lost consciousness.

I've got the hospital report from that night.

I take the piece of paper from on top of the amp and begin to read.

01:35 AM: Consultant Dr Roberts arrived. Estimated blood loss: one litre;

01:37 AM: Vaginal examination by Dr Roberts. Fully dilated LOA at spines, 1+ caput (that's just where the baby is inside Sarah);

01:38 AM: CTG brady (that's for bradycardia, which is really bad). Five minutes. Decision for delivery in room as both theatres still occupied. Neonates called and present in room;

01:39 AM: Manual rotation of the head;

01:40 AM: Forceps applied and locked with ease;

01:41 AM: First pull. Good, decent;

01:43 AM: Second pull;

01:43 AM: Episiotomy (that's a cut at the bottom of the vagina). Head and baby delivered. Floppy and white-looking;

01:44 AM: Cord clamped and cut and baby handed to paediatricians;

01:45 AM: Resuscitation commenced;

01...

Sarah lost five litres of blood that night. Five litres is all we have. She has more than ten different people's blood in her now.

Sarah lived.

Tom died.

I go back to the loop pedal and start the music. It is Music Two, quite quiet.

Spoken:

And that is where leave Sarah and Emma and James and Tom.

I'm sorry that Tom died.

I'm sorry that Tom dies.

I tried to find any pathway where…but that's not the shape of this story.

Cos I don't want to live in the universe where Tom dies, I want to live in the universe where Tom lives. I want to live in the universe where Icarus lands on his feet I want to live in the universe where Orpheus doesn't turn around. I want to live in the universe where Verona has email.

But we don't. Our experience of existence can be so painful and there is no panacea for it. We are so fragile. Suspended from the finest thread between birth and death, a snip away from oblivion.

Music One gets louder.

Sung:

But if we sing
Sing like it is the first time
Then nothing bad has ever happened to us

Music Three.

Spoken:

And the thing is: stories never actually begin or end, it's just where we join them or leave them. So if we go forward in time: four years from now, six years after Tom died, enough time for wounds to heal and yes, six years is a long time but they are big wounds and they'll knit themselves together into scars that are stronger than the skin was before and yes they'll hurt, they'll really hurt when it gets dark and it gets cold which is why it's so important that we keep each other warm with our kindness and with our care and with our friendship.

Music One gets louder.

Sung:

If we sing
Sing like it is the last time
Then nothing bad can ever happen again

Music Three.

Spoken:

So we're four years in the future, six years after Tom died and James and Sarah and Emma and Lydia are going to get into a car and drive to the sea because in two years' time Sarah and Emma are going to adopt a little girl called Lydia and we're going to take her to the sea for her birthday. I'll drive and we'll sing her the song that you sung for her before the show.

Music One.

Sung:

The world is so big and we are so small,
And sometimes it is hard to make sense of it all,
But I love you and I'll be here,
And one day Lydia we'll go for a beer

Spoken:

Now what I'm about to say might sound a lot like a greengrocer telling you apples are fundamental to your humanity because I'm a story teller and I'm telling you that stories are fundamental to our humanity, whether they're stories that happen for real out there, or stories that happen for real in here, whether they're the stories we tell ourselves or the stories we tell other people, they're all true when we believe them.

Sung:

And if we sing,
Sing like it is the first time,
Then nothing bad has ever happened to us

Spoken:

Stories continue.

Sung:

And if we sing,
Sing like it is the last time,
Then nothing bad can ever happen again

Spoken – the following text is looped over the top of the song that has played before:

Okay. Stories then. There's the oldest story, the story that God made humans in his image, now I don't believe that, I believe we made him in our image, which is why he's such a fucking dick. Or foxes, I put my own narrative on the fox in this show. I decided that it wasn't my buddy but it could have been because foxes have fifty per-cent mortality every year and half of them die on the roads. Or rainbows, I love rainbows because their story has changed for me as I've grown up because when I was a kid I thought they were symbol of God's promise that he wouldn't flood the shit out of us again and then I grew up a bit and learned in science class that they're actually pure light, refracted into its component parts but now I know that they are a symbol of love and pride and the fight to be yourself in a world that doesn't want to hear that but they're all true and we get to choose the stories that we want to.

The loop crescendos to an unbearable volume.

I'm definitely going to do a cartwheel.

I do a couple of cartwheels.

The loop stops.

Thank you.*

---

* A footnote at last! Sorry if you've missed them. *Revelations* is a new show. What you see when you come to it will be different from what is written here. Turns of phrase will be more elegant, the progressive imagery will be better integrated and jokes will be there (or not, who knows). It's currently at about the stage *A Hundred Different Words for Love* was before all the changes in the footnotes and appendices . I thought about registering that at the beginning but I've noticed that people will take whatever one says at face value. So if I'd have apologised before you'd begun you would have naturally thought less of this. Probably. You might be great and immune to such blandishments.

James puts on a song ('Everything is Awful' by the Decemberists).

Anyway. Thank-you for reading this book, it's a work in progress, but as my friend Tom Bell says: aren't we all. Now go and hug a loved one and then tweet me about it @jdsrowland. I feel incredibly lucky to have been let loose on a book. I thought this sort of thing was done by other people. Well done if you got this far, your prize is absolutely nothing. After all, you can't win fun can you? You can only have fun.
I'll never see you again.

WITH THANKS TO:

Charlie Covell   Dan Goldman   Tom Hall

Paul Flannery   Tom Bell   Wiggy Cheung

Andrew Gruen   Stewart Pringle   Johnny Chiodini   Amy Fleming

Will Young   Jonny Donahoe   Paddy Gervers

Dean Rogers   Lauren Mooney   Jess Clark

Kyle Ross-Richardson   Jon Cooper   Neil Connolly

Kat Bond   James McInnes

Jess Mackinnon-Patel

Tim Robinson   Emmanuella Bredaki   Ben Attwood

Isley Lynn   Camilla Whitehill

Holly Morgan

Bec
Boey

Tom
Moores

MIRIAM
ATTWOOD

Mim
Black

Stephen
Myott-Meadows

Joseph
Brett

Lizzy
Jewell

Roann McCloskey

Brid
Kirby

Rhik
Samadder

Alex Wolpert

Richard
Rogers

Rosie
Collins

Matthew
Rowland

Hannah
Storm

Giles
Havergal

Lucy Briggs-Owen

Mark Trend

Ben Moor

Alice
Lacey

Milly
Thomas

Serena
Grasso

George
Spender

Appendix I

HOW WE MAKE THE SHOWS

I've been friends with people who self-generate material and make their own shows for a long time and thought I should do it too. I talked and planned over and over but never actually made one. There seemed to be some invisible barrier to my magically generating a work ethic, I was utterly paralysed by a blank page and it seemed like writing just wasn't going to be something I did.

Then in January 2015 I'd just finished doing a play with Daniel where he let me improvise a fair amount. I then had an absolutely terrible year. No acting work at all and a very big break-up (in quantity of time and quality of pain). I needed to something to fill the void and that is how *Team Viking* came about. The fact that half-way through making it, just as I was losing momentum, Vault Festival programmed it gave me a necessary boost but it really did take that extraordinary cluster-fuffle to get me to make it.

I had an idea for a story and rather than discussing with anyone and everyone (in the pub) as I had before, I only talked to Daniel about it and asked if he'd make it with me, which turns out to have been the best thing I have ever done professionally. I then spent several months researching and thinking of ideas and doing very little tangible work. Dan asked me how I was getting on. I said 'nowhere' and he suggested that I just tell the story to him. Just go round to his house and get through it (he has since done this with many other solo show makers and insists on calling it a 'sesh' to everyone's distaste). The prospect of doing that made me feel incredibly exposed, it was horrible, I was terrified that there was no substance to the story, that it'd last about twenty minutes and would be bad.

It was really bad. However there were a few good bits, it felt fine to do and lasted eighty minutes without even getting to the end. It wasn't cathartic in the way that sketching out an idea over several pints always is but it was tangible. It made me want to do it again and better. So I did, and again and again. Every time I recorded it and listened back over and over and it improved. This is how all three stories were made.

The most crucial factor is people. I always deliver them to a friend or two; the very act of trying to amuse and move one of my incredible friends is the thing that has made the stories worthy of anyone's time. (I always present the victim(s) with wine before I start because I know how bad the improvisations are and I'm not a monster.)

I have a rough script by January (I didn't for *Revelations*) and then rehearse with Dan and turn it into something proper in time for Vault Festival in the first week of February. They then sit dormant until July when we do a bit of re-rehearsal for Edinburgh. The first ten days of Edinburgh feel like the biggest learning curve and the shows seem to settle a bit after that.

Team Viking has done a national tour and I learned a good deal more about the show through that. I'm certain that *A Hundred Different Words for Love* will do the same. The journey has only just begun for *Revelations* with Edinburgh still three months away (I haven't even written it down yet, although by the time you're reading this I will have done for this book). I hope you enjoyed reading three shows at different stages of development.

I highly recommend anyone struggling to get words down on paper to just say it out loud to someone you trust and admire.

I was having a writing day with the wonderful Isley Lynn recently (I'm new to writing days but apparently they consist of chatting quite a lot, drinking lots of tea and occasionally writing, they are the best) and she suggested that it doesn't matter how I make the shows, that generating the words for a show makes a person a writer. I'll take her word for it.

Appendix II

These stories and therefore this book would not exist without Daniel Goldman. It's an incredibly close relationship, the closest working relationship in my life. He's been there for the days where it was all breakthroughs and the days where I sat catatonic.

Logistically the shows do not make any money until they tour therefore Dan has worked with me for about two months a year for three years for absolutely no money. Ha. Terrible.

Thing is though, I'm not really sure what Dan has done. I know it's been vital to the shows but the ant knows nothing of the microscope nor the mouse its laboratory (although I hope they occasionally have an inkling they're being fucked with).

Thankfully I'm far from alone in making a one person show and a long way from unique in having a very close relationship as a writer/performer with a director. I asked a couple of my heroes (who I'm lucky to be friends with) about their work partners. This is Ben Moor writing about Erica Whyman:

'Her eye is exceptional, and not just theatrically – she knows what to say in a mentoring way too. She's a spirit-lifter. And each production displays her tip-top skill and judgment in stagecraft. A solo show can be rehearsed by the soloist in an empty room, but there's no energy given to it by a fourth wall; a great director brings a new life to something that may have become drained by a year of over-work. Erica has been an essential collaborator; she always notices moments of bad structure in my pieces, and is brilliant at creating the tempo of the finished production. She is also wonderfully calming as the show enters the crucial phase of technical rehearsal and final dress runthrough, when I tend to despair. Even an hour with her can make a show a thousand times better…'

Ben has a more classically theatrical approach to making his shows than I – he brings a fully finished draft to Erica before they work together and the dramaturgy she provides is less a discrete role and more a function of her direction. Saying that, everything Ben has described applies to Dan.

Milly Thomas wrote of Sara Joyce with whom she made the play *Dust*:

'I don't actually think I could have made work without her. The thought of the show has made me balk multiple times. I approached her by sending a poorly written fart of an email that had a vague treatment and a couple of jumbled scenes and a concept. You are completely vulnerable in those moments between pressing send and the reply. The replies become all important and she immediately was able to straddle the gap between the personal and the professional. It's important to get on with someone. Especially when your subject matter is autobiographical and or personal, intimate. Telling stories can be a messy business. But you don't have to be their friend. I think that's very important. Sara is director/dramaturg. That's a hugely exciting and terrifying position and a huge amount of faith to put in the other. She is doula and midwife. There's a practical and holistic process going on at the same time. We agree 80% of the time. That 20% for me is often where the magic happens. We weren't friends before making the work and now I'd take a bullet for her. We met in the work.

It means you can begin with a dispassionate eye and develop a shorthand. The clinical builds to the nuanced and textured. The whole thing is a trust exercise and balancing act. She is as much the work as me. When you make work people are often trying to make things 'through' people. Everyone has a creative vision and while a producer dictates the course, the director of a solo show has to steer that ship. You are at your rawest, most vulnerable and yet, somehow, your most empowered.'

I think Milly has said everything that needs to be said there. There are two specifics that stands out though: 'You don't have to be friends' and 'I'd take a bullet for her.' There is something in the relationship that requires and enforces closeness.

Chaos theory suggests that a butterfly flapping its wings in Hydrabad can cause a hurricane in Hawaii and Dan's influence pervades the stories not just for the huge structural changes he has suggested but also for the quiet and gentle acts of kindness that have allowed me the space to make the shows. Although that phrasing is difficult. We make the shows together, they are our shows but they are also my shows. I think that's the crux of our relationship – Daniel has the grace to work through me.

Like I say, I dunno.

Thanks Dan.

Appendix III

BY DANIEL GOLDMAN

Occasionally we get asked how we make the shows...and there are various answers, I suppose.

Practically, we've made these shows through improvisation. The first thing we do is get into a rehearsal and with no further preparation, I make James tell me a story – the story. The only rule being that he has to keep talking for an hour without stopping. The theory being that the story will take care of itself and it is the story that will carry James through rather than James carrying it. Telling a story for an hour is really hard. And if you don't believe, give it a go. Try to tell a story for an hour and you'll see how hard it is...except that what happens is that if you don't allow yourself to stop or give up, and you're able to still continue, then suddenly a depth of detail starts to emerge and weird tangents pop up and new memories come to the surface and so suddenly the constraint becomes liberating and the story gains in texture and depth and richness. All I'm trying to do is listen, just listen and receive and write down everything that grabs me. It could be a turn of phrase. It could be a little story or an anecdote or one of those weird little tangent. It could equally be a well judged pause. Or silence. Or reference. And so James tells me a story for an hour and then we talk about it for the next two. I look through my notes and repeat back to James what I liked, what made me perk up, what made me laugh, what made me stop writing. Essentially, this first improvised go at the story becomes the template for the show. It becomes very clear where the heart of the story is and where the story wants to lead the audience. We talk this through, I give James my notes, he takes them, and we go and have lunch. Having done this one hour improv with me, James then goes off to do a whole series of improvs to friends. Having done those, and asked each friend for their thoughts, James and I come back together and the actual crafting of the piece begins. But again, pretty much always through hour long improvs. A classic rehearsal session for us will be a cup of tea, followed by an hour-long improv, then another cup of tea and notes... and then sometimes another hour-long run. We do do some structural dramaturgical work which involves moving bits of the story around, mostly to do with playing with time, but most of the time, we just do these hour-long runs, then notes, and then James goes home and writes a bit more. Once we've sort of worked out how the story works, then we'll incorporate the music...and that's all James being brilliant.

All of that gets us to our first performances in front of a paying audience. Which is a super important step because that's when they tell us what they think and we discover the truth about what's funny and what's moving etc. All I do when we do those first performances is watch the audience and listen to them. When are they bored, when do they hold their breath in, when do they laugh and why etc. We take all of that on board, and then, perhaps this might seem strange, we sort of leave it to one side, as we continue to work. It's useful of course, but more useful is working out what we've felt during those performances. You can't pander to an audience. You have to stick to what you believe... And the improvs and the runs continue.

One thing we've found incredibly useful as we've gone on is to record every single hour-long improv. With pretty brilliant recording technology in every phone and every tablet, it's become very easy to record everything we do… and often we'll come back to a previous recording to see if in run seven say, we did a particular bit of the story in a more interesting way. I'd recommend it to anyone making a solo show. If technology is used in sports to improve performances, why not do so with the arts. Anyway, sidebar over, we will do twenty, thirty runs together as we craft the show before we're happy that the show is ready. This allows us to get a real sense of the piece as a whole. How it works rhythmically, where it drags, where we need a musical interlude etc. It works for us…but it requires a lot of trust.

Which leads me to my other answer. The other way we make the shows is through shed loads of trust and patience and tea in James's case and coffee in mine. It's a slow process. It's very un-British in that sense. We spent a good six months making *Team Viking*, four or five on *A Hundred Different Words* and three on *Revelations*. We've spent a lot of time together. A lot of time not actually rehearsing or writing but just hanging out, talking about the show, chatting through notes. Given the materials we're dealing with and the stories we're telling, there has to be a lot of trust and care and kindness in the room. As James has alluded to in his other post, more than anything, it's a question of being present. Present in the room…and present in each other's lives. The stories are ours. That's how it works.

Daniel Goldman

Appendix IV

I have been very fortunate and had a couple of lovely months at the Edinburgh Fringe with *Team Viking* and *A Hundred Different Words for Love* (what will occur with *Revelations* remains to be seen) as a result of this, a fair amount of people have asked for advice. So I thought I'd pop it down here in case it's useful.

The most important advice I have is this:

Work out what the worst case scenario is and figure out if you can live with that. It can always happen regardless of how well prepared you are. Resilience and luck are crucial.

My friend, the wonderful comedian Kat Bond put in a good word for me at Just the Tonic on the same day another performer pulled out so I got a space. I'd never thought I'd actually write a show or be able to take it to Edinburgh despite it being on my horizon for a long time. So just trying to make each day as good as possible for whoever was there was enough.

Team Viking played to audiences of between two and fifteen people for the first two weeks of Edinburgh in a room with two lights and a woodworking class above it. It was tough. Numbers picked up as a result of word of mouth and a few encouraging reviews but I really think that the reason both of those things happened was because I was still enjoying performing the show.

I get more people in to shows regularly now but I still check on whether I'd find it crushing to perform to an empty room again – if I would then I'd have to think seriously about stopping because that would mean I don't care enough about the story I'm telling for the show to be good or successful.

My cousin Miriam happens to run one of the best PR companies around (Storytelling PR). None of our family have ever been involved in theatre so this is probably the most ridiculous piece of serendipity that has assisted the shows. I think having a good PR is now almost necessary in order to have a 'successful' Edinburgh, which is difficult (sorry Mim) but by no means an unfair expense.

I don't flyer because I'm bad at it, but I have reaped the rewards of good flyering for my shows (especially at Summerhall). Try and make sure that a flyerer has seen your show and likes it before they try and get people in. Pay them well.

Financially I'm privileged and that has made everything possible. I was very fortunate in 2016 to get a job that allowed me to earn well so I saved enough money to write off the expense of Edinburgh. If serious poverty could have been the result of not making money from *Team Viking* I would never have been able to concentrate on the show. I say this to register the limits of my advice. It's disgusting that just being a part of Edinburgh in any way requires a lot of money and it's the responsibility of everybody in the industry to address this stupid inequality.

Be kind.

I'm not sure if I've mentioned this elsewhere but there is this tricky phenomenon that doing the right thing often makes life better and so doing the right thing sometimes makes me worry that I'm just being selfish and mercenary.

Doesn't stop it being the right thing though.

You set your own parameters of what is successful. Set achievable targets. Don't rely on anyone (be it critic, peer or audience) giving you what you want, they might, but expecting it will inevitably lead to disappointment. Make sure you have friends around in person or on the phone to have good times with because there is an infinite supply of happiness far more important than any show.

Appendix V

ARTWORK

The shows are very aural (lol) if you come to see them the most visually arresting image you are likely to see is me putting on a hat or lighting a match or taking my clothes off (granted the last one is less arresting than it is capital punishment).

However, we live in a visual world and anyone doing a show has to provide artwork for posters and flyers. I think that having a good image for a show makes a big difference as people almost certainly see a shows picture before they see the show. A good image will encourage people to buy a ticket, a bad one may stop people.

It has turned out that the pictures have influenced the shows far more than you might expect, they certainly influenced them more than I thought they would and the shows are now indivisible from their images. I thought therefore they were well worth a little explanation.

TEAM VIKING

My friend Rosie Collins is a remarkable photographer and a very dangerous drinking companion. The idea for this photo, standing in the Thames in a funeral suit, holding a flaming torch made of flowers emerged almost fully formed into my head. The plastic viking helmet was absolutely a part of that hazy image but I think Charlie actually suggested it before I said it out loud because she is quicker than me.

I'd hoped that I would have been in the river off one of the Thames' low tide beaches but like the lackadaisical legend I am, I neglected to check when low tide might be. So instead we did it on the steps down outside the National Theatre because it was high tide. We waited for security to wander away but we needn't have bothered as quite a crowd gathered as we started to work. I used a can of Lynx to get the paper flowers to light. I also only had two bunches, which meant Rosie only had about thirty seconds to get this picture. That's how good she is.

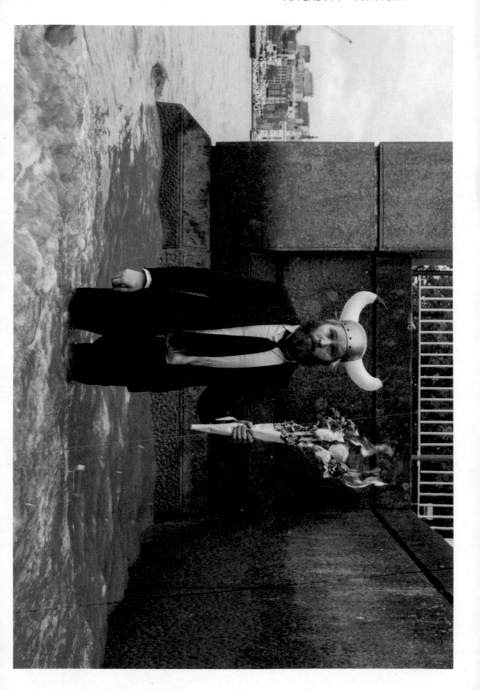

A HUNDRED DIFFERENT WORDS FOR LOVE

The *Team Viking* picture had been good and I didn't want to try to replicate it... So, instead I thought we should invert it, not landscape, portrait, not in day, at night, not wearing a suit, wearing a dress, not standing in water and holding fire, but standing in fire and holding an umbrella as it rains. Certainly a much more impressionistic image and one I had to justify with the show – the image was absolutely the reason for me wearing a dress.

My very talented friend Joseph Brett (more an animator than photographer but good at more or less anything) was around and also has together with his partner Bec an allotment and therefore somewhere we could make a fire for me to stand in.

The way we made it look like I was in a fire was by making a line of fire in front of me and then one behind. Bec stood on a ladder with a watering can for the rain (which was just as well because without the sprinklers the dress and I would have definitely caught fire).

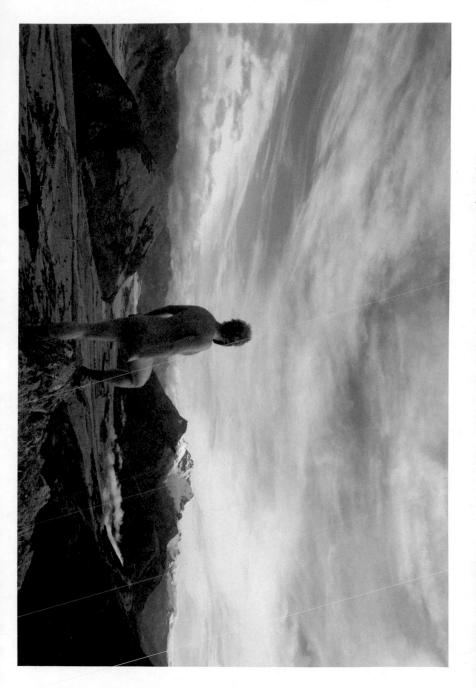

173

Appendix VI

R ight. So. Obviously I've been having a bit of fun, making up lies in the footnotes. I'll explain why I did all of that. I think it's worth saying, but I don't want to be patronising so do feel free to just not read this.

Team Viking is not true. None of it. It can't be because I'm summoning up feelings in the present in the show that I cannot possibly feel in the present every time I do it.

Team Viking is true. All of it. It has to be because I'm summoning up feelings in the present in the show and it only works if I feel it in the present every time I do it.

Tricky.

I find it a bit weird when people think that a work of art is more valid because it's a true story… I also think that doing creative work is important. Here is my argument attempting to justify my job, how it doesn't neglect my social responsibility. For stories to work you have to get people to imaginatively engage with them, for them to fly the audience has to empathise. Imagination and empathy are like muscles, the more you use them the stronger they become and I think that most of the problems we have in the world would be solved if everybody exercised empathy. None of that is the same as directly helping someone who needs and wants help. Wonderful, soul hammering art – far greater than anything I'll ever make – has existed for millennia and hasn't yet knitted together the open wounds that exist globally. I just hope that I'm proffering a bit of collagen.

I don't think that fiction is better than documentary work (although I generally like it more). I just don't believe that one is more real than the other (hence the meta-structure of *Team Viking*).

Some people have been quite cross about my saying 'All of it is true' when most of it didn't happen, in fact a really good theatre that I really admire were going to program it and then changed their mind when I told them that the story wasn't true. I was obviously upset about this at the time because it's never pleasant to feel misunderstood. The fact is though, they didn't misunderstand me, they just didn't like the show, which is fair enough.

I'll quickly tell you what really happened if you're interested (if you've got through the screed above you deserve something).

Essentially everything up to and including the Christmas Pudding story is true. Everything after that is made up. That's it really, my dad's dead, my ex-girlfriend broke up with me in an incredibly patronising fashion and my grandad immolated a festive dessert. I have been incredibly lucky that so far in my life I have not lost a single one of my brilliant friends. I'm very lucky.

Oh yeah, and Tom and Sarah don't exist.

Sarah is an amalgam of every kind, good bit of my friends but especially Charlie Covell and Tom Hall.

The childhood sections of Tom are based on my childhood friend Richard and his more grown up self is every flash of charisma and chaos in my friends distilled into a form perhaps not dissimilar to someone who will remain nameless.

I've said this at the end of the show a couple of times:

'So this is the first show in a trilogy, in 2017 I was just about to perform the second story – its sequel called *A Hundred Different Words for Love* which draws quite a lot on feelings I had in breaking up with an ex-partner. I was on the phone to my childhood friend Richard (who used to come around to my house when his mum went out on dates) and I was explaining how I was worried I might upset my ex by mentioning things connected to us. Richard responded: 'I wouldn't worry about that, Jim, after all *Team Viking* was all about your grief for your dad and nobody knew that did they.' I didn't say anything for a long, long moment. I hadn't realised. I didn't know. I asked all my friends who had seen the show and been around when Dad died. I asked my mum, I asked Daniel who I make the shows with. Everybody knew except me. They all thought that I knew. It goes to show doesn't it: Stories are funny things.'

I don't think the show has anything to do with the relationship I had with my father, it's about my friends. In a way the show is inspired by the grief I experienced in losing Dad but I think that's only a sliver of the story's heart.

There is nothing either good or bad but thinking makes it so.

Appendix VII

A HUNDRED DIFFERENT WORDS FOR LOVE:
PATHS UNTAKEN

Shakespeare had every word (and more) to shape his sentences and he set down sonnets, Beyoncé had innumerable arrangements of both her body and her body of work; she created her Coachella set, Michelangelo looked at a block of marble and saw David.

I am at least as good as them.

There's been this thought that occurred to me a while ago and has changed the way I look at every bit of art (I subscribe to Seiriol Davies' opinion that art isn't a compliment, it's just a type of thing). It came from anxiety about being misunderstood. That every piece of work shares a characteristic – it is the thing that the maker or makers decided to create over every other possibility.

So now I always bear that in mind, the chips of marble on the floor, the subjects untouched, the paths untaken.

Here are some of the old bits that didn't fit well into footnotes:

'It was funny as well having the example of Sarah and Emma going on the same time because they just, they didn't overthink. They'd only been together six months before getting engaged. They hadn't worried, they just went, okay. Come on then, let's do it and there was I, incapable of even getting past simple words.'

'…with the fact that we'd both had things before. Not in a day to day tangible, jealous way, that stuff was great, she was frank from the first walk, she mentioned an ex-boyfriend, the ice was broken, it was very easy to mention all of that, not during sex obviously, but after, we'd rate each other's performance based on our ex's. No. That was never weird. The thing I struggled with…'

'It was wonderful being around Sarah and Emma through that time as well, they were like our big sisters, showing us the trail ahead, like, 'When you grow up you'll be like us and get married and it'll be great.''

'We didn't break up because she was sexually assaulted which she was while we were together. A guy at a bar, grabbed her, touched her, kissed her, someone she works with… I'd like to say that my first reaction to this was anger, fury at him but it wasn't. It was jealousy. I don't say this to excuse myself, just to register my reaction, that it's always possible to be a dick, it's always important to try hard not to be.'

'Sarah, my oldest, oldest friend was not that fussed by the idea of the wedding. Emma was the one who was really into it. The main thing for both of them was 'we want to spend the rest of our lives together, isn't it cool that as two women we can now get married' but Sarah wasn't fussed about the day, Emma wanted a proper party so that was the plan. It was cool helping them for me and the girl because it was like playing grown-up. Talking about how amazing it was, me and the girl decided that when we got married (in imagination land, based on the way we talked about it) when...'

'It was funny because with me and the Girl, when we talked about it – we did talk about the idea of getting married but it always felt removed, imaginative, a speculative exercise in intimate chat. I think it might be because I'm quite a mindful person (buzzword) in part because of my job and I've been very lucky all through my life to be present, to be in the moment. With the girl at that point, with our lives, weekends away with Sarah and Emma. It was bliss. Just enjoying that. Those moments. Days of endless kindness. Looking back on it now, I was setting myself up for a fall but it felt like just embracing the embrace of the moment.'

Appendix VIII

REVELATIONS: GETTING NAKED

I knew I'd be taking all my clothes off in the show as soon as the thought occurred. The images were of a part of that but it's also the logical conclusion of a set of stories that strip me metaphorically. Penises are problematic. I worried about it for all kinds of reasons but the top two were body image and it becoming the talking point of the show. The former has so far been absolutely fine – it's the right thing to do for the show and I'll definitely die one day so my shame may live on after me but I won't be there to care. The latter remains to be seen (as it were).

My wonderful friend Rhik Samadder decided to write about the experience of me getting my kit off better than I could. Rhik and I have bonded over many years of appreciating the weirdness of the world so his article about my penis being published in the *Guardian* is in some ways an audacious act of one-upmanship that I will struggle to better.

In a stunning act of duplicity he was very liberal with the facts. So I would like to make it clear that I have never used the phrase 'truly vulnerable in the room' (although I agree with all the things my friend has invented me saying). Also, I gave him two comps, he has never paid for a show in his life.

The fact that he made the same Chekovian reference as I do sometimes before the show is a complete coincidence (I recorded the show he came to and didn't do that bit). 'Chekov's Penis' is a funny thing to say. He didn't write the headline.

COLUMN INCHES:
MY VISIT TO SEE ANOTHER MAN'S PENIS

My friend James wants to show me his penis, under an arch in Waterloo. I'm pretty sure, anyway. He's invited me to a piece of work he's performing at the Vault theatre festival, which features full frontal nudity, and is a one man show: I've done the maths. I find myself vaguely worried. Maybe it'll be like the film *There Will Be Blood*, which doesn't have that much blood in it. But something about the phrase 'full frontal nudity' doesn't trade in ambiguity. I'm hoping I won't have to drink up his milkshake.

Anyway, it is a brave thing for anyone to do, breaking the taboo of public nudity. I want to support my friend, but also find the whole thing quite funny. 'What time do you un-trunk your junk? Is it the climax of the piece? Why r u doing this' I message him. 'I knew from the beginning the process would involve nudity,' he replies. 'As a white, cis-gendered heterosexual man, it's the only way I can be truly vulnerable in the room.' It's good he's thought deeply about this, but it does sort of ruin my fun.

My puerile attitude may be masking my own discomfort. The playwright Anton Chekhov wrote a famous dramatic rule, that art should never contain distracting or superfluous elements. He used the example of a gun, visible on a wall in a play's first act. 'If it's not going to be fired, it shouldn't be hanging there.' It's fair to say I have similar concerns.

The idea of the phallus looms large in our collective consciousness, representing the power and worst urges of the patriarchy. Violence, arrogance, sexual aggression. I'm terrified of it too. It's easy to equate men with their penises, forgetting the problem lies in their brains, not their pants. The actual appendage gets a bum rap. As the owner of my own modest pipe, I'm aware these notionally intimidating organs can be functional, funny, or almost cute, like a sleepy anteater. The discrepancy is like the scene in *The Wizard of Oz* where the curtain is drawn away to reveal the wrinkly, puce old fool working the levers. You? You're running the show?

As we take our seat and the show begins, I wonder if the experience will change our relationship. How could it not? With me is a friend, whom I have only told one thing about the evening, and who genuinely asked if this was a strip show. I'm nervous for James, and for me. I start to worry about size comparison. Where does that come from? Outside of porn, male genitals are hidden in our culture, giving them an outsized significance. Exaggeration and anxiety both flourish in the dark. No one habitually texts their partners 'You're gonna get some of this average penis, baby, during our statistically normal lovemaking.' But wouldn't that be more helpful?

I shouldn't have worried. It's a wonderful piece of theatre, charming, inventive and alive. When we finally reach dong o' clock, the moment is not only totally earned, but carries hefty emotional weight; the logical culmination of a plot strand both hilarious and heartbreaking. 'All art contains a didactic element, and to earn that right, the performer must be ultimately exposed,' James later explains over a drink. I wish he'd stop talking, because he's ruining it. All I know is, I've never seen a penis better deployed. The piece, fittingly called *Revelations*, is playing again in March, before a national tour. You should check it out. The show, I mean. I'm talking about the show.

Rhik Samadder
First published in *The Guardian*, 12 February 2018